Stay Young and Vital

Stay Young And Vital

by
Bob Cummings

GROTON PRESS, INC.

74 THIRD AVENUE   BROOKLYN, NEW YORK

To my Mother, Reverend Ruth Cummings and my Dad,
Charles Clarence Cummings, M.D. Physician and Surgeon

TABLE OF CONTENTS

Chapter 1. LET'S START LIVING 1

Chapter 2. ARE YOU FULLY ALIVE? 13

Chapter 3. WONDERLAND NUTRITION 19

Chapter 4. THE TOP OF MY FORM 25

Chapter 5. THE MYSTERY AND MIRACLE OF YOU 35

Chapter 6. YOU ARE WHAT YOU EAT 44

Chapter 7. "SEVEN RULES FOR FLYING HIGH" 60

Chapter 8. VITAMINS FOR VIGOR AND VITALITY 67

Chapter 9. MINERALS ARE A MUST 76

Chapter 10. HANDLE WITH CARE 82

Chapter 11. POSITIVE HEALTH 92

Chapter 12. FADS, FACTS, AND FOOD VALUES 103

Chapter 13. ARE YOU LOP-SIDED? 121

Chapter 14. POSITIVE LIVING 129

Chapter 15. MAKING THE MOST OF YOU 140

Chapter 16. YOU AND YOUR PERSONALITY 151

vii

Chapter 17.   SILHOUETTE CONTROL   159

Chapter 18.   SEX AND SALAD   167

Chapter 19.   THE TIME OF YOUR LIFE   174

Chapter 20.   HOW TO LIVE LONG—AND
                LOVE IT!   185

Chapter 21.   TURKEY WITH A RIBBON   190

Chapter 22.   TAKE CARE OF YOU—FOR ME   202

Introduction

For a little over fifty years now I've been adventuring and experimenting with this thing called Life. And I've reached at least one firm conclusion. It's this: The most important and the most unselfish thing you or I or anyone has to do in this world is to *take care of number one!*

That is what this book is about—how I believe you can take the best possible care of you.

I've never met a man or a woman or a child who didn't instinctively want to be as healthy, vital and attractive as possible whether they were ten, or thirty, or fifty, or seventy, or ninety. I've come to believe honestly that the instinct is there because the possibility is there—that there is a simple, common sense way by which we can stay at the top of our form at any and every age.

"Taking care of number one" to me is not the guide line of the selfish egotist but rather the dedicated task of Divine Selfishness, because taking good care of you is really complete unselfishness.

Is that difficult to believe?

If you are as attractive as you were meant to be it is true that you will have a happier life. But so will the people around you. You'll be decorative at the office. You'll adorn the kitchen. You'll be so nice to go out with—or come home to.

If you are at the top of your form, health-wise, your disposition won't prickle and irritate either you or those who pass your way.

If you or I are full of energy and enthusiasm we are of more value in our work, in our homes, in our country. We are better citizens. We use our leisure more creatively. We can't help being better friends, better parents. And we don't run the awful risk of becoming a burden to ourselves and others. We've all seen examples of extreme *misguided unselfishness,* parents who have sacrificed their health for their children who in turn have had to sacrifice their lives caring for invalid, aging parents. That is only one outstanding warning to all of us to *take care of number one, or practice Divine Selfishness.*

When *you* take care of *you* first, nutritionally, psychologically, spiritually and financially you are so much more able to positively take care of others—to be of service—as well as to enjoy your own life. And service to others, of course, is a number one prerequisite to success, good fortune, perfect health and happiness—all of which we want for ourselves—so the Divine Selfishness which fits us to serve others in turn brings us what we most desire.

Now the question is, exactly *how* do we take the best care of number one—ourselves?

In giving you my personal answers I want to remind you, as they do in all the books, that my conclusions are my own, but they've worked for me and for my guinea pigs (see acknowledgments) as well as the converts I've made en route to the half century mark. For further authenticity I'm going to carry you through some phases of my progress—the Protein Me, the Vegetarian Me, the Lop-Sided Me, which led to the fourteen common sense rules for positive health, and the four basic rules for dynamic living you'll find detailed between these covers. I firmly believe these eighteen rules, if you *use* them, if you live *them,* can help *you* to attain and maintain more vitality, more enthusiasm, more zest and attractiveness, more harmony of mind and body, more love of life and success in living it starting right *now,* than you have known before.

They have worked for me.

They have worked for my family, and many of my friends.

They can work for you.

Remember, your well being is not only important to you, not only important to the people who love you or who depend on you, but because we are all one great family, one great unity of intelligence and effort, what one does affects the whole. Your well being is important to me.

Or I could phrase it differently.

I, personally, could say to you, personally,

Take care of you for me!

ᴥᴥᴥᴥᴥ

Let's Start Living

A friend of mine once met a magazine writer who had been assigned to "do" a Bob Cummings story. "Well," said my buddy, "when you meet Bob, don't be surprised if he's lying in a reclining chair writing a book or reading his script through periscope glasses and munching reindeer meat."

This is not true.

I almost never recline.

Of course, I've never written a book before, either.

But scripts I know about—scripts I read. And every motion picture script begins the action with the magic words, FADE IN. At this point the actor knows that he is about to meet his invisible audience for the first time. Since this is my first experience with writing a book I assume that when I type PAGE ONE, CHAPTER ONE, I have, in a manner of speaking, magically FADED INto your life. You and I have been formally introduced in a literary sense. But if instead of this invisible meeting I had the magic to transport you onto my set or into my living room, if we could meet face to face, instead of finding me on my back peering at you through periscope glasses, the scene would go something like this:

FADE IN:
   INTERIOR CUMMINGS LIVING ROOM—DAY
   TWO SHOT CUMMINGS AND GUEST (YOU)

              B. CUMMINGS
             (rising from sitting
             position on an ordinary
             couch and extending hand)
   I'm Bob Cummings. How are you?

              YOU
             (returning handshake)
   I'm fine, Bob. How are you?

             B. CUMMINGS
             (very happy)
   I'm fine!

Now that isn't brilliant dialogue but it's exactly the way it would play if we were nice, well-bred people—which we are. Now supposing we were *honest* people as well. Would our lines still be the same? If you said, "I'm fine," could I believe you? When I said, "I'm fine," would you believe me? Would you believe that I feel exactly as vital and energetic and excited about living today as I did ten years ago (and if you were to make it twenty years ago I could honestly say I feel *more* vital and energetic).

If you were actually listening and did believe me—and you would have every reason to, because it's the truth—you might react in one of three ways, and I would know a lot about the state of your health from that reaction. If you were really feeling "fine" we'd hurry over the greeting and go on immediately to other things. You'd take it for granted that I was on top of the world. If you felt sick or sickish, aging, aching, or paining, you'd probably resent any bounciness on my part (and when I feel fine I have a tendency to bounce). You might even take it all as a personal insult or enjoy discussing your poor health. If, on the other hand, you were not quite sure *how* you felt, if you didn't feel "fine" and you didn't feel "awful," just in between, with the weariness and the worriness and the acid indigestion, you'd be a little embarrassed and try to make a joke of the whole situation.

How do I know? Because I shake hands with a couple of thousand folks a month and that's exactly the way they behave if they don't go through the ceremony automatically. The joking kind are the most common. I'll illustrate the technique.

That Old Tired Feeling

Last week I walked into the studio and ran straight into an actor I hadn't seen since our early days on Broadway when we were both young leading men. We went through the handshaking routine and read the lines as laid out above —except that he already knew I was Bob Cummings. Then he looked me over. He suddenly realized I meant that I felt "fine." That embarrassed him so he said: "I hear you are on a health kick," by which I assume people mean that I am interested in feeling fine all my life—which I am—so I nodded.

"I read something in a magazine the other day that would give you a chuckle," he said jokingly, prodding me in the ribs. "It was right up your alley." I resisted prodding him back because he didn't look like he could sustain it and then, since I wasn't due in make-up for fifteen minutes, and I hadn't seen him in a long time, and I thought he might be frustrated all day and go on wearing that expectant grin if I didn't, I gave him the verbal prod he was waiting for.

"Tell me," I said meekly.

So he told me this story which he swore was true (but I do not!) about a young man who consulted his doctor because he was in exceptionally good health. He felt fine. He could tear a telephone book (the Los Angeles or New York directory) with his bare hands. He arose each morning with the sun and couldn't wait to get to his rowing machine. At the studio he was making more enemies than friends by doing the day's work of two men before lunch.

And he didn't like it!!

Since he was no longer depressed or morose he felt his temperament was deserting him and he missed that familiar gloomy feeling—the days when he was grumpy and critical and hated everybody. It had been weeks since he had beaten his wife. A cheerful sunshine dazzled a world which he had been accustomed to view through dim pessimistic lenses— and this whole cataclysmic change in such a short space of time—at a very early age—all without dying and going to heaven.

His friends had begun to regard him as a freak and he was inclined to agree with them.

The good doctor sought hard for scientific clues and finally uncovered three: (1) the man's wife had been going to nutrition classes and actually revamped their diet; (2) together they had been attending church and the minister had persuaded them to do some mental and emotional house cleaning; (3) they had been reading the Bible and were beginning to pray.

Now the diagnosis was sure. The patient was suffering from an acute attack of Man-As-Man-Should-Be. The symptoms were obvious: Excessive health. Joy and serenity. Abundant energy. And the cure? Simple. Just a return to the old ways of eating and thinking, and an immediate curtailment of prayer.

"Gee, Doc," said the relieved patient. "You don't know how grateful I am. If you could only get me back to normal —if I could only get that good old tired feeling again I'd ask for nothing more."

"Don't give it a thought, my friend," said the kindly physician. "Follow this advice and we'll have you feeling worse in no time!"

Now, my old buddy obviously thought the joke was on

me—and I had to laugh. Partly at the story, which was good satire. Partly at his delivery. He's a good actor. And partly because it's my secret hunch that the joke was on him.

He knew that I, too, had just celebrated my fiftieth birthday. What he didn't know was that his yarn had confirmed an idea I had had that night that maybe I'd like to write a book about how to feel fine.

To celebrate that fiftieth birthday I had planned a gay evening. I discovered that some of my friends thought we should hold a wake.

To me the half-century milestone marked the beginning of a lot of new, exciting adventures, the opening of a tract of unexplored territory.

To them it marked the beginning of the end.

It had taken me a part of those fifty years to become convinced that the natural condition of man—Man-As-Man-Should-Be from birth onward—was healthy, joyous, attractive, energetic. And I had given a lot of time and study to working out a way of life by which I thought this state could be achieved.

Now, at fifty, was I willing to concede that it was all a joke or a delusion? That if you didn't gallantly laugh off the half-century mark you had to weep instead? Or had I actually proved in my own life that you could and should "feel fine," that you could and should start living more vigorously at twenty-five, fifty, or seventy-five, by following some sane, sensible rules?

Well, the place to answer those questions was to take a look at my own life. Was anything I had learned worth passing on? Had I proved anything at all?

Man-As-Man-Should-Be

As a pilot I knew the advisability of having my aircraft checked every fifty hours. As a man who had lived approximately 18,250 days or 438,000 hours, not counting leap year, it seemed a good idea to run a fifty-year check on Bob Cummings.

What sort of condition was he in?

How had he functioned in the preceding twelve months?

Was his system for getting the most out of life as valid at the half-century as it had been at thirty or forty?

Well, B. Cummings had been going at a good clip day and night over the past year—directing his own television show, acting in it, making personal appearance tours, flying his own plane—so he seemed to be functioning on a full schedule. As to condition—no illnesses, not a cavity in his teeth for years and years, no need for glasses, full crop original hair, waist line steady. Check! And on over-all attitudes—how did he feel? Great! Energy? High. Vitality? No decrease. Enthusiasm? Boundless. Problems? Plenty, but feels able to cope. Love of life? On the increase.

Check complete and satisfactory. B. Cummings all set for another fifty or hundred years or more. (God willing!)

Now, did all this make me a freak? I didn't think so. Did it make me in any way outstanding or remarkable? Again, I didn't think so. To me it seemed more natural than "that old tired feeling." Was it something to set me apart or swell the size of my hat-band? Definitely not. All it did was indicate that, at this stage of life, I was still a Good Animal. Obviously an animal that can't sense danger and protect himself is prey to all attackers; if he can no longer hunt he'll have a tough time making a living in any jungle; and if he's too lame to keep up with the pack he's left far behind. The chances are he won't survive long.

But there is no reason for the human animal to begin to drop behind the pack at forty or head for the scrap heap at fifty. I have discovered in my personal experience that you are never too young to feel a hundred percent better than you feel right now, and never too old to regain the symptoms of Man-As-Man-Should-Be—health, joy, enthusiasm, attractiveness, energy! And the exact methods, which have worked for me and which I have seen work for untold others from teen-agers onward, will be detailed in this book.

But first I'd like to do a little ground work.

Be Your Age—And Proud of It

Let me start by saying that I, personally, don't hold with the cult that worships Youth. In fact I don't hold with any cults or fads (having had some experience with them in the course of my life, as you will discover as we go ahead). My feelings on this matter were very well expressed in a story told by General Vandergrift of the Marines. It seems a patient came to one of our field hospitals with the complaint that he was unable to sleep at night. The doctor advised him to eat something before going to bed. "But, Doc," the patient reminded him, "two months ago you told me never to eat anything before going to bed." Standing tall in his professional dignity the physician replied, "My boy, that was two months ago. Science has made enormous strides since then."

And so it is. For a while everyone takes square pills and walks in the night air. Then suddenly only pear-shaped pink pills have potency and night air turns poison. My feeling is that we should accept with gratitude what science establishes as *fact* but refrain from chasing every rainbow theory—or thinking that the only pot of gold worth finding at the rainbow's end is Youth.

I am *not* young for my age. Heaven forbid! I hope I'm *right* for my age. To me the goal is to *be your age and be proud of it!* To be the most attractive, useful, productive, happy thirty—or forty—or fifty—or sixty—that it's possible to be.

Some of the most dynamic and successful people I know waved a cheery farewell to the youth of the twenties and thirties and went intelligently on to rich, mature living—

Gloria Swanson, Perle Mesta, Sophie Tucker, Eleanor Roosevelt, to mention only a few on the distaff side. And on the other, Cary Grant, Jim Stewart, John Wayne, Gary Cooper, in my own profession; in sports, Slammin' Sammy Snead, the great golfer who at forty-seven had the best year of a very big career; or in politics, Senator Theodore Green of Rhode Island who, at the age of ninety, gave up tennis but not legislating.

On the other hand, too many people wilt early or die young, just as they should be beginning to live. Yet the secrets of physical fitness, attractiveness, productivity, enjoyment, dynamic living, for male or female, at any age, are not really secrets at all! They are laws authored and endorsed by a Divine Hand. They can be proven by anyone who will take the time to learn them and the trouble to live by them. These are the laws we will discuss in future chapters. But the first step is to see what we have accepted as true—and what the truth really is.

Max Mueller has said: "All truth is safe and nothing else is safe, and he who withholds the truth from man for motives of profit or expediency is either a coward or a criminal or both." So let us, being neither cowards nor criminals, search for the truth together.

To begin—is it true that we were meant to be well, healthy, fully functioning, whole and wholesome, from our entrance to our exit on this particular stage?

Do you believe that it can be done and that we were meant to do it?

Too many people, in my experience, do not. They accept deterioration and decay of teeth, eyes, etc. practically from birth. And at the half-century-mark they are incredulous, astounded, and even offended when, for example, they check up on my appearance, vitality, and age. And they do check, bless 'em. After all, the professional actor is beholden to his fans—those lovely, wonderful fans, without whom he has lost both his market and his reason for acting. I have found that the actor is as much on display as the meat or fruit or vegetables in a super-market. Most every actor has been inspected and poked and prodded and felt on public appearance tours with the same impersonal appraisal used by a good housewife in selecting a roast or an avocado, until they reach the point where they would like to say wistfully, "Look, you are *my* fans. Do I always have to be just *your* actor?" and do some prodding themselves.

Once a pair of elderly ladies approached me, walked around me, nodding and chattering about me as though I were an inanimate object. Suddenly one leaned forward and smartly pinched the skin of my fore-arm the way you would pinch a peach to test for ripeness. She looked interestedly through her glasses as the blood receded and the skin turned white, then beamed as it returned to the afflicted area with a rosy glow. "Good circulation," she said cheerily to her companion and off they went, satisfied with the actor animal, without even a kind word for Bob, the man. I sincerely hope it boosted my box-office rating by two because I wore a black-and-blue mark for several days.

Some of the youngsters are more personal. They will get very close and remark to each other with satisfaction, "Look, no wrinkles." Or, "How about that? Not a gray hair!" Then I feel as if I'd been awarded a junior Emmy or Oscar.

Some, however, comparing my age and physiognomy, simply say "freak!". Some say "how?". And some, like one little lady who approached me at the stage door after a personal appearance, came right out and said, "How dare you?" Her point was that the Bible definitely stated that "the days of our years are three score and ten"—seventy, to be exact and modern—and according to her reckoning any man who wasn't at least beginning to go to pieces at fifty was uncooperative if not downright sinful.

This attitude is fatal if we are to make the effort to achieve that other ideal—what I have called Man-As-Man-Should-Be.

Is this limitation the little lady wished to impose actually a law? Or simply a mood line by a magnificent poet which we have made a law by our own acceptance of it?

Back to Methuselah

Generally speaking the Psalms in the Bible are full of comfort and hope and joy. It's in these songs that we are offered the symbol of the Shepherd leading his flock beside still waters, making them lie down in green pastures, and the loving promise He makes the individual sheep, "with long life will I satisfy him. . . ." In between these promises of hope is inserted a doleful tune—the 90th Psalm—in which the writer, troubled by God's anger and wrath, by his own sense of sin, announces our life expectancy as "threescore and ten." Now, were we to take this as Gospel truth, to accept it as a heavenly order? Or to regard it as a transient emotion of the Psalm-singer?

If we are going to search Scriptures for the answer we are in for a great surprise, for we will have to go back to Methuselah, back to Genesis, where we find this venerable gentleman living nine hundred and sixty-nine years—his offspring, Lamech, to seven hundred seventy-seven—and Noah lived nine hundred and fifty years despite the flood.

The Bible proudly states: "There were giants in the earth in those days" and "the daughters of men were fair." This was a pretty nice state of affairs surely, and they had every right to be proud of it. We begin to wonder what subsequent civilization introduced that served as giant-killers and maiden-dimmers. What reduced us to a seventy-year span and Bottled Beauty? I think you'll know the answers before you've come to the end of this book.

Don't misunderstand me. I'm not sure I want to go back to Methuselah. Nine hundred and sixty-nine years might be too much television even for me—but I am convinced that the life span of each one of us should be thrice seventy, at least! That the average human being on earth probably lives only thirty-three percent of the period God intended for him, and that we can all do something about it immediately.

Why Die When You've Just Learned to Live?

Yesterday I read in the papers of the death of a prominent young scientist—at forty-six. And that *is* a young scientist. And just last week three members of my own profession left us suddenly but finally, one at thirty-eight, one at forty-seven, the other at fifty-one. All four of these men had lived just long enough to harness and train their individual talent until it was completely developed. A talent matures slowly, through study, self-discipline, experience. The scientist, the educator, the actor, the legislator, I could go on through the entire list, doesn't reach full usefulness much before what we call middle life. Before that it is being perfected, polished, nurtured. Does it seem logical that a Divine Intelligence would develop a shining lance to place in the failing hands of a body ready to collapse? Would you think it anything but a shameful waste, a needless loss and sorrow, to see an apple tree come into full fruitage just as the trunk and limb powdered into dust?

It should not be so and it need not be so! And we, this minute, can begin to change our thinking about it. If we are not convinced, let's look at the record: Titian painted his masterpiece, the "Battle of Lepanto," at the age of ninety-eight. Verdi wrote his great opera "Otello" at seventy-four, and "Falstaff" at eighty. Kant, at seventy-four, wrote his "Anthropology." Root, at eighty-four revamped the World Court. Edison built chemical plants after he was sixty-seven. Sarah Bernhardt was acting until her death at seventy-nine, even after losing a leg; General MacArthur was supreme commander of the occupation in Japan in his seventies. Chaucer's "Canterbury Tales" were the composition of his later years. They were begun in his fifty-fourth year and finished in his sixty-first. Sir Christopher Wren, the great architect, retired from public life at eighty-six; after that he spent five years in literary, astronomical, and religious pursuits. Thomas Hobbes published, in the eighty-seventh year of his life, his translation of "The Odyssey," and the following year "The Iliad." Dwight Eisenhower was keeping the rigorous schedule of President of this country after his seventieth birthday, becoming our oldest President, and still a golf expert.

And these examples of the intended harvest from the ripened years also bring me to my second point: people believe that, if they lived two hundred and ten years, the last hundred and fifty would be spent being pushed shakily about in a wheel chair and this, for sure, would be a horrible state of affairs. But it should not be true at all!

By the time we scan the Bible from Eden to the Exodus and thence across the wilderness, we find Moses only lived to be a hundred and twenty—still it clearly states that at this exalted age "his eyes were not dim, nor his natural forces abated."

~~~~~~~~

Chapter 2

Are You Fully Alive?

A great many people who think they are fully alive are in reality one-third or two-thirds dead already—and this includes teen-agers as well as their parents and grandparents. I think that's probably what was in the mind of a certain clergyman when, lying fatally ill, he decided to send a farewell note to his vestrymen. He wrote:

> Go tell the vestrymen I'm dead,
> But they need shed no tears;
> For though I'm dead I'm no more dead
> Than they have been for years.

The average human being today, unlike Moses, has his "natural force abated" practically from birth onward. We aren't actively ill, but we aren't well, either. We are operating at about fifteen percent of capacity both mentally and physically whether we are aware of it or not. That "old tired feeling" becomes so natural we accept it as the norm.

Laziness, for example, considered a sin among our grandparents, is today more apt to be a deficiency disease suffered just as easily by the teen-ager who sits in class on an empty stomach as by the senior citizen whose conditioned attitude is that he has "earned the right to jest set a-piece" and dunk doughnuts while he disintegrates simply because he is sixty years old.

Are We Healthier Than Grandma and Grandpa?

There is a rumor around that we are an enormously healthy nation with a great life expectancy and that we are far, far healthier than our great-grand-dads were. But is this so? This has been a very controversial subject recently and statistics can be interpreted many ways. In an interesting pamphlet by V. Earl Irons, called "Your Life," he answers it thus:

"All the propaganda and so-called proof (that we are healthier than our great-grandparents) is based upon the fact that the Life Expectancy figures of Insurance Companies show that your great-grandfather's life expectancy *on the day he was born* in 1850 was only 38.3 years, while your boy born a hundred years later in 1950 had a life expectancy *on the day he was born* of 68 years. Since the life expectancy has increased thirty years, almost double, it is simply taken for granted that as a nation we must be healthier collectively and individually than our grand-dads. Actually what do the Life Expectancy figures show and mean?

"Here are the Life Expectancy years for various ages for 1850 and 1950, a hundred year spread, per Government census and Metropolitan Life Insurance Company releases:

> "As of 1950—
>
> "A new born baby could expect to live 30.1 years longer than his great-grand-dad on *his* birthday in 1850.
>
> "A ten year old boy could expect to live 13 years longer than in 1850.
>
> "But a forty year old man could expect to live only 5.2 years longer.
>
> "A fifty year old man could expect to live only 3.1 years longer.
>
> "A seventy year old man could expect to live only 1.6 years longer."

Dr. Norman Jolliffe in the New York State Medical Journal, September 15, 1955, put it this way: "Although in America the life expectancy at birth is near the best of any civilized country in the world—at the age of forty life expectancy is near bottom."

The great benefits health-wise over the last hundred years have been to reduce infant mortality and death by contagious disease. But while these have been reduced the deaths from degenerative diseases have increased 44 percent. (Degenerative meaning "change in the chemical constitution of the intimate cells of a tissue from a higher to a lower form" —such as tooth decay, heart trouble, hardening of the arteries, and even cancer. And with this type of chronic illness you can drag around only functioning on two cylinders for some time before you are aware of definite symptoms of disease.

In a report on the Health of the Nation by W. Coda Martin, M.D., this is borne out by medical experiment. Said Dr. Martin: "A check-up of five hundred apparently healthy business men, average age of forty-eight years, at the University Hospital, Ann Arbor, Michigan, revealed that 41 percent of them suffered from physical diseases of which they were not aware, and 11 percent were aware of some specific illness or a total of 52 percent who needed immediate treatment, and 77 percent of these healthy men had some physical abnormality which did not require immediate treatment."

In other words, by and large, they just weren't ill yet, but they just weren't well either.

Let's Wake Up and Look!

None of this presents a pretty picture—and there is more to come. But it is vitally necessary, if we are to make a serious effort to follow the suggestions in succeeding chapters, that we first know the truth about the situation with which we are dealing.

This is not a matter of telling anyone how to look younger

or have sparkling eyes, or catch her man, or reinterest the
girls. This may be and will be a delightful side benefit. But
the urgent, important reason is that we must wake up to
our present condition and determine here and now to become fully alive, fully wholesome, fully useful, which in turn
will raise us to a level of happiness we have not known before.

It is a serious situation. Dr. Martin tells us that as early
as 1939 chronic diseases had replaced acute infectious diseases to such an extent that Dr. S. S. Goldwater, Commis-
sioner of Hospitals in New York City, warned that if its
prevalence continues, "America may some day become a
nation of invalids."

And with chronic diseases the prevention—always easier
than the cure—lies in your hands and mine.

Degenerative conditions are no longer confined to older
people. The over-all picture of health in the young man of
draft age is rapidly deteriorating as revealed by the draft
rejections from World War I to the Korean conflict, over a
short period of thirty-two years. In World War I, 1918, 21.3
percent of drafted men were rejected and 9.9 percent were
placed in a limited service group, or a total of 31.2 percent
were not physically able for active military service. At this
time the physical standards were high. In World War II,
1941-1943, the total found unfit for military service despite
reduced physical requirements was about 41 percent. The
rejection rates increased sharply with age. The total percentage of rejected men from age 38-44 years was 64.7 percent. In the seven years from June 1948 to June 1955 some
52 percent of the young men called for pre-induction examination were rejected for physical or mental defects—an increase of 11 percent over World War II, or a total of 21
percent increase in rejections since 1918 in spite of marked
lowering of the physical standards.

A condition that is often considered a minor problem

and does not get much publicity, according to Dr. Martin, is allergy. But to 20,000,000 Americans who suffer with these very annoying symptoms it is a major problem. Probably one of the greatest economic problems (and the most annoying to the individual, no?) is the "common cold." A Gallup Poll in 1954 disclosed that 18 percent of the population were victims of "colds" every month, or a total of 18.8 million. In one week period ending December 11, 1954, a survey by the American Institute of Public Opinion found colds reported in one-third of American homes with an estimated total of 29,000,000 persons affected. Nation's Business Magazine, January 1956, reported that the American sneeze cost billions. We spent $1,000,000,000 on tissue alone. (This comes as quite a blow!) It is estimated that American business loses $5,000,000,000 annually from the common cold.

A medical examination of fifty executives revealed that fatigue was an outstanding complaint of 60 percent of the men. Nor is weakness and fatigue confined to the adult. The result of a muscular fitness test of American children between the ages of six and sixteen revealed that 57.9 percent failed a minimum muscular fitness test. Dr. Martin made a further interesting statement in commenting on a recent nutritional report from a ten-year survey on the eating habits of the present day teen-agers, which would give us an idea of "what to expect in the next twenty-five years." The survey found approximately three-fourths, or seventy-five percent of boys and girls between thirteen and nineteen under-nourished.

And this in America . . . the land of plenty!

That is going to take some explaining. And we will get to it in a later chapter. But this is a sad picture, going from bad to worse, and it vitally touches on you and me. We must see that this rapidly deteriorating sufferer described is not, *cannot* be, man created in God's image and likeness, Man-As-Man-Should-Be by Divine decree.

We must now believe that we were meant to be well, healthy, whole, wholesome, and happy, and that if we are not, something can be done about it and *we are meant to do it*.

In this frame of mind come adventuring with me.

Chapter 3

Wonderland Nutrition

Socrates said: "Know thyself."

He probably wasn't the first, and he certainly wasn't the last to present this challenge. Physicians, psychologists, ministers, parents, and pals are urging it on us one way or another most of our lives. The great adventure, I think, is to take the dare, to discover what makes us tick—the flaws as well as the limitless possibilities wrapped up in our personal package—and find a way to keep ticking harmoniously at the top of our form, useful and happy, without unnecessary time lost in suffering physical and mental breakdowns and costly repairs.

My dad issued the first formal invitation I received to "know myself." Since he was a doctor his emphasis was on nutrition and a sound body—as sound as God could create and man maintain it. I have discovered since that many people shy away from this particular facet fearing "narcissism" or "hypochondria" or some other long name for what they interpret as vanity and self-centeredness. This is too bad because the object is neither to be constantly checking the body for imaginary flaws nor to fall in love with our own reflection, but to make the most of the equipment God gave us as a free gift. To me it seems a spiritual responsibility.

St. Paul, in writing to the Corinthians, said: "Know ye not that ye are the temple of God, and that the spirit of God dwelleth in you? If any man defile the temple of God, him shall God destroy; for the temple of God is holy, which temple ye are." (1st Cor. 3:16-17)

That puts it up to us squarely, and while it may seem harsh at first glance, good sense gives us every evidence that, when we break God's laws for maintaining the temple in proper order, even through ignorance, it does degenerate and is eventually destroyed. I had a friend once, a dear, kindly, devout little lady, who believed that God was "visiting" her with bodily pain and suffering, who prayed loud and long that He put her back into running order, while all the time she went on violating every basic, impersonal health law. I don't think she ever knew a *well* day in her life, but she accepted this as God's will for her with a martyr's smile while stubbornly refusing any responsibility for maintaining at a functioning level the instrument He had given her.

She refused to be healthy if she had to do anything about it personally—and she rationalized this attitude until she thought it saintly.

Kahlil Gibran, the great Syrian poet, glimpsed this personal responsibility when he saw the body as "the harp of your soul," and we have already discussed how the waste saddens us when the instrument rusts or disintegrates just as the greatest music is ready to be played. Agreeing with the poets, that sound and practical fisherman, Izaak Walton, wrote in *The Compleat Angler:* "Look to your health; and if you have it, praise God, and value it next to a good conscience; for health is the second blessing that we mortals are capable of—a blessing money cannot buy."

If the wisdom of the ages doesn't convince you, there's always the authority of common sense—although I will confess that when I first plunged in earnest into the world of nutrition, I thought perhaps sense would never again be common. It was a little like falling down the rabbit-hole with Alice and landing in a topsy-turvy Wonderland.

Getting to Know Myself

In the course of my personal adventures I have been, variously, an engineering student, an Englishman (with an accent and pedigree), a Texan (but not a Texan of distinction), a singer in the Ziegfeld Follies, a pilot (in war and peace), an actor, director, professional prevaricator (both on and off the screen, the phony heir to a goldmine, and a vegetarian.

Obviously, all this while I was experimenting.

I have lifted weights, done every conceivable kind of exercise, eaten yards of roots, grass, and dried seaweed, made my way through Scotland on a one-cylinder motorcycle and a minus zero budget doing "tongue-grooves" by the wayside, and perpetrated a show business fraud that was not discovered until I was forced to expose it myself in order to make a living, all of which is part of the story of how I personally got acquainted with myself and is bound to unfold as we go on.

At one point, years ago when I was Deanna Durbin's leading man, my zeal surely exceeded my common sense as well as the sage advice of the publicity experts. With another devout vegetarian I would march around the studio lot singing a devout vegetarian song which, if I remember correctly, went something like this:

> "Roots, fruits, and nuts,
> Muscle, speed, and guts,
> We're the guys who eat no ham,
> We eat no beef,
> We eat no lamb—
> We're vegetarians!
> Rah! Rah! Rah!"

You can easily see why, looking back, many of my adventures had the fantastic quality of Alice's Wonderland. Here, too, were Mad Tea Parties where folks sat cheerily with

March Hares, Hatters, and Dormice, trying to draw treacle from a treacle-well. Life was full of little bottles inviting DRINK ME, the contents of which would shrink us to ten inches, and small cakes labeled EAT ME which would cause us to shoot up until there were once more giants in the earth. Mushrooms had to be carefully inspected to see exactly how and where they were grown, for, as the Caterpillar told Alice, "one side will make you grow taller, and the other side will make you grow shorter."

All of this I investigated. It took a lot of years before I was able to sort it out and set it into sensible simple rules that worked for me. At one time or another I could quote various authorities who truly took opposite sides about the same mushroom—or meat, or starches, or any vegetables. One authority said it was good for you and the other that it was bad for you, until the only possible answer seemed to be to give up eating entirely, and in my confusion I most certainly would have accepted this easy, economical solution if some authority had also told me how to get rid of my appetite.

Oscar Wilde claimed that "experience is the name everyone gives their mistakes," and you can see that I've had a lot of experience. However, through trial and error—and the inevitable mistakes—I came to some basic, common-sense, conclusions.

The Conditions That Prevail

The first one is: *That we are the most over-fed and undernourished nation in the world.*

I know this is a horrifying statement in view of our wealth and scientific achievements. I know too, that it sounds very impersonal because we think of a nation, even our own, as "they"—those others—while it is really "we"—you and me. This means that there is every chance that you and I, our children, our friends, our older relatives, are eating *too much of food that isn't doing a good thing for us.*

Most deceptive of all is the person who looks excessively well fed, the one who in less polite circles might be called fat. Such a lady climbed on the scales in our market the other day and two grinning urchins craned their necks to watch the big wheel go round. The scale, however, was on strike and only registered a paltry eighty-two. "Can you beat that?" my wife heard one exclaim to the other. "She's hollow!" He didn't know how right he was. While we may be neither over or under weight, nor actually ill, we are probably not healthy either, and won't be unless we educate ourselves and do something to correct the situation. Let's look at some facts.

A primitive Masai warrior in far off Tanganyika looks forward to a healthier life with less chance of dying of a sudden heart attack, a longer life providing he can avoid death by contagion or accident (and who is willing to debate the relative danger of a predatory lion and the same instincts in a modern motor car?) than a thoroughly civilized, carefully tended Wall Street tycoon. The Masai has better teeth, better vision, is stronger, taller, his muscular tone firmer, than the usual local bank manager.

The Masaï belle, dressed simply in a length of sacking and decorated with a profusion of coiled wire, has whiter, evener teeth, more sparkle to her eyes, a sounder body, a happier disposition with less chance of nervous or female disorders than the cherished wife of a Washington diplomat or a bejeweled movie star.

An average adult Eskimo (male) who has lived isolated from civilization can carry a hundred pounds in each hand and a hundred pounds in his teeth. While this is no entree to Park Avenue society nor a recommended method for making your first million in these United States, it yet demonstrates the Eskimo as a Sounder Animal than the head of the civilized household who folds under the burden of carrying the family's weekly washing. And among the jungle Indians of the Amazon the women just naturally have a straight spine and noble carriage duplicated in our society only by the ex pensively trained professional model.

If I now say that all of this is chiefly a matter of nutrition I can hear some of my readers shout, like the Queen in Wonderland: "Off with his head." And some say, as the Mock Turtle said to Alice: "Explain all that." While the remainder who remember that I've promised to recount some adventures, say with the impatient Gryphon: "No, no! The adventures first, explanations take such a dreadful time." I think I'll decide for the "adventures first" because from them came the explanations, and if I can make the explanations clear I may win my case and my head will stay on my shoulders—where I have become very attached to it.

Chapter 4

The Top of My Form

It was inevitable that I should be aware of the care of my body even as a kid. Dad, a physician and surgeon, graduate of Rush Medical College in Chicago, was one of the most remarkable and forceful men I ever knew—a conscientious and dedicated doctor twenty-four hours a day. He habitually washed his hair and hands with tincture of green soap, even at home, to be surgically clean and prepared for the emergency of a sudden accident. He was constantly in training for an operation (any operation) and I can remember his sitting in our living room reading a book with sutures and Lysol solution in a bowl beside him, a rubber glove on his right hand, tying and untying knots in the sutures using only the fore-finger and thumb, to keep his fingers sensitive and supple. He could do it equally well with his left hand.

Far in advance of his time on matters of nutrition, Dad was all ethics and no collection, with little of the diplomat to temper his approach. He was perfectly capable of telling a wealthy patient all set to pay liberally for pink pills and sympathy, "there's nothing wrong with you physically except that you aren't getting the right things to eat." And even that was more tactful than the methods he used at home.

His early advice to me was: "You've got to run as fast as you can in this world to stand still—and if you've got to run you'd better get the right fuel. Don't eat slop!" It wasn't very elegant. He didn't mean it to be. He meant it to be effective and it was, for I can still hear the words ring in my ears all these years later. It was effective with mother, too, because I can remember when he was trying to educate her nutrition-wise and she put something on the table of which he disapproved, he would scowl and remark, "That's slop!"

Of course, he didn't have all the facts and fancy words to work with that we do now, enzymes, amino acids, vitamins and so forth. None of them, in fact, were known when my father started preaching nutrition. He had two words in his nutritional vocabulary: *slop*—the negative, and *protein*—the positive. It was from my father that I first heard this magic word, PROTEIN, a word we'll meet again and again in this book. *"You are protein,"* said my father (and he was one-third right, as we shall see). He not only tried to educate the family and his office patients about proper food, but when he and mother, now a convert, helped build the Jaspar County Tuberculosis Hospital located in nearby Webb City —and by help I mean assisting in pouring concrete and laying tiles—father insisted that the hospital have its own farm on adjoining acreage, its own dairy herd, its own eggs and poultry. "We'll feed 'em back to health," he said—and did!

When I was about eighteen my father went to Chicago to attend a medical convention and there met a fellow nutrition-pioneer. This meeting had a direct if specialized bearing on the second phase of my adventures in getting to know myself physically, because after dad came home I got an intimate working acquaintance with my tongue, soft and hard palates, larynx, esophagus, hyo-glossi muscles, and vocal chords—all the odds and ends pertaining to my voice—and discovered that they, too, were protein.

All this came about because (a) while I was sound of wind and limb, I was too quiet a teen-ager to suit my father (imagine!) and (b) my father had an avocation to which he was almost as dedicated as he was to his vocation. His relaxation was singing. A beautiful tenor voice had helped him through medical school when he got odd jobs as a "super" complete with tights and spear in the Chicago Opera Company and he kept this interest alive in conservative Joplin by discarding the tights and joining the Presbyterian choir in the church across from our house at 520 Pearl Street.

At that Chicago convention he heard a lecture by a German-trained throat specialist, Dr. Eugene Feuchtinger, who spoke on the health of the vocal apparatus as it pertained to nutrition and use. The vocal apparatus, said the lecturer, was made of *protein*, and you couldn't expect all those delicate little chords (a veritable harp) to function properly unless you fed them the proper stuff. Naturally these two protein pioneers, Drs. Cummings and Feuchtinger, fell upon each other with great enthusiasm.

When it developed that Dr. Feuchtinger tested his theories as a voice teacher and conducted the Perfect Voice Institute of Chicago, which had an extension course in book form, father decided this was just the present to bring home to young Robert.

"It's the very thing to bring him out!" he explained to my mother. And it did just that. Under father's prodding eye I studied the written manual which emphasized the fact that it took fuel to run the complex vocal apparatus. Proper eating, therefore, was basic. Then too, there were silent exercises called "tongue-grooves" which I mastered and practiced vigorously. Sometimes, with the exaggerated enthusiasm of youth, I did as many as twenty-five-hundred of those in one day—nobody ever did so many. And then there was the actual singing. For this phase my guidance was entrusted to a friend of my father's, one Percy Pither, who conducted the Episcopal choir.

And so I studied how to feed my vocal chords, and wiggled my tongue, and sang for Mr. Pither and it certainly served to bring me out of myself, for it not only helped me develop a very durable speaking voice, but later on I became a singer in the Ziegfeld Follies and you can't get much farther out than that. To make my living as a singer was more than a triumph for a quiet guy, for I was not gifted with an exceptional voice such as my father had. But I got away with it. Here a small talent, properly cared for and developed, got me a big job which is more exciting, to my way of thinking, than a big talent rusting in a closed throat.

Actually, however, I was "brought out" before my Ziegfeld days and the process of getting a foothold on the New York stage was so engrossing that I abandoned any interest in nutrition for a spell. It was easier and quicker to eat like everyone else did; during the depression it was nice to be invited to eat just any old carbohydrates as long as they were free—and on the road with a show the greasy spoon was the most convenient. I thought I was too busy getting ahead for what I considered side adventures—so I understand very well the problem and thinking of the Young Adult, which we will deal with more specifically in Chapter 19.

My dad died just after I opened in my first Broadway play and there was no longer anyone to insist on the difference between "slop" and "protein." I continued with my "tongue-grooves" until the momentum of habit simply expired and that, temporarily, seemed to be the end of getting to know myself nutritionally. Then a year or two later I met up with some vegetarian folk who sold me on the horrors of eating flesh. Like all half-informed people, I was nicely receptive to food-fads. I knew just enough from dad to realize that nutrition was important but not enough to chart a sane, sensible course for myself. Once convinced that there might be something in what these folks said—willy, nilly, I gave up eating meat.

The Vegetarian Me

For eight years I belonged to the ranks of the vegetarians and fruitarians and a rare mixed-up world it was.

Carolyn Wells described the condition of the fruitarian very well in this limerick:

> "Miss Minnie McFinney from Butte,
> Fed always and only on fruit,
> Said she: 'Let the coarse
> Eat of beef, and of horse,
> I'm a peach and that's all there is tutte."

Obviously the fruitarians are not vegetarians but sometimes the vegetarians aren't either. There are degrees in the lodge. Some famous vegetarians like George Bernard Shaw supplement their raw carrots with liver extract and both he and Mahatma Gandhi were free with dairy products, eggs, cheese, milk and such. The simon-pure vegetarian scorned these things as well as nuts, grains, and fruits. The results too, were uncertain, for while vegetables inspired such writing geniuses as Shaw and such political and spiritual geniuses as Gandhi, the ranks included slightly over-dressed bearded hermits and slightly under-dressed nature boys as well as members of the Muscle Brigade, none of whom produced much of anything.

Some had religious convictions. Some were motivated by a pure and burning zeal for health. Others, like myself, had mixed emotions, in my own case centered around a shuddering aversion to pictures I had been shown of slaughter houses and ill-preserved meat. Illogically I recall that I was particularly moved by the thought that spices and condiments first came into demand in Europe to cover the odor and flavor of badly preserved meat—forgetting that this was well before the day of even the old-fashioned ice man.

At any rate, for some years my experiments seemed to prove that I was on the right track. My general feeling of well-being increased. My tendency to colds decreased. I felt valiant while on the road with plays as I pioneered and struggled to stay true to my cause, no small consideration then for while today when the science of nutrition is growing up stores and restaurants are provided for the neophyte or initiate, in those days it was a battle to hold the vegetarian standard high away from home base.

A year after adopting my meatless ways I found myself at the Cohan-Grand Theater in Chicago as leading man with the Ziegfeld Follies feeling very fit and in good voice. My songs ran from the delightful sentimental "A Pretty Girl Is Like a Melody" through the sophisticated "I Like the Likes of You" to the nostalgic Americana of "Home on the Range." Moreover I was traveling in star-studded company, a cast that included Fanny Brice, Eve Arden, Willie and Eugene Howard. So pleased was I with myself that I contacted the Perfect Voice Institute hoping that Dr. Eugene Feuchtinger, my first singing teacher, would come to sit front row center and admire this apt pupil. The old doctor, however, like my father, was gone, but his son, another Eugene, came to hear me. We met under odd circumstances, since I was at that time carrying on one of my great impersonations (to be detailed in a later chapter) and I don't know how impressed he was with my voice. I do know that he wasn't too impressed with my vegetarianism although, short of reminding me that I was *still* protein, he didn't say much.

Seven years later out in Hollywood, California, I wasn't too impressed with it either!

I began to believe I was a better singer than I was a vegetarian. Or possibly I knew more about the one than the other. For by 1940, after some years in the motion picture business, I had discovered two things. One, that I continued to have a weight problem. Vegetables do not contain a very high percentage of protein in relation to their bulk and it's protein that burns up the fat. Furthermore, I just couldn't chew up enough lettuce and parsley and celery to appease my appetite and I had to reach out for more starch than my system would have demanded if I had been getting sufficient protein. The second factor was even more important. Somehow, after struggling through acres and acres of vegetables I still did not have the drive, the vitality, that I needed for successful living.

The fully informed vegetarian today may know how to get all the things his body needs, but obviously, I did not. In that one year, 1940, I made nine pictures only to wind up on the verge of collapse. Under pressure I simply did not have the stamina required. *The proof* for me, was not in eating the vegetarian pie, at least not the way I baked it. And so, after eight faithful years in the club, Rah! Rah! I resigned. I simply began to eat meat again. It was a good thing, too, for I was about to get into a meat eating outfit—the U.S. Air Force.

The Protein Me

During the next few years Uncle Sam took charge of my diet and I ate the *plat du jour* recommended in the Air Force. The only nutritional adventure worth reporting came just before my discharge in 1945. For the first time in my personal history I lost my appetite. This is a physical phenomenon beyond the control of the ablest physician or biochemist, common to the male animal when he falls in love. And that is exactly what I did.

On week end from Muroch Flight Test Base toward the end of the war I had gone down to Hollywood and run into the famous photographer, Paul Hesse. Paul was wildly enthusiastic about my meeting a "wonderful, beautiful" young actress, Mary Elliott, under contract to M.G.M., who had just been risking her pretty neck entertaining troops from Greenland to the south Pacific. Not only was she "wonderful and beautiful" according to Paul, but she was different. "She isn't overly impressed with Hollywood but Hollywood is impressed with her," Paul chortled. She was, he said, the slightly aloof and "very unattainable" product of a fine old southern family, and quite a product on her own as well, managing to keep her sense of values in the sophisticated world of make believe.

"You've talked me out of it, Paul," I said sadly. "I can't handle anything that elegant on Air Force pay." But I did meet her briefly at a party and she certainly *looked* "wonderful and beautiful" and she surely *was* "unattainable" because I got one smile and then was shoved to the edge of the crowd and never made it back as far as the ten yard line.

A short time later under orders from my C.O., Colonel (now General) Clarence A. Shoop, I flew a group of performers assembled by the Victory Committee from Hollywood to Muroch to do a show. As pilot I didn't see the performers and, as passengers, the performers didn't see me so I had no way of knowing that the "beautiful, wonderful, unattainable" Mary Elliott had unwittingly entrusted her pretty neck to my care. We met literally "on stage" after the performance at Muroch when Colonel Shoop introduced us to the audience together. And that was when and how I lost my appetite. Nor did I regain it dietetically. "Slop" or "protein" were equally uninteresting. It wasn't until some months later after Mary and I were married at the Fliers' Chapel in Riverside that I even seemed to remember that normal people ate three meals a day.

Our wedding was a delightfully family affair for my mother married us (and the effect on me of my mother becoming a minister plays an important part in the discoveries I want to share with you later.) At any rate, our marriage has gone on being a family affair, what with five young Cummings now out of the nursery, the eldest bucking for the Air Force Academy. Script and director credits for the entire performance and casting of "My Life with Mary," or "I Become a Family," are still sharply contested by our good friends, Paul Hesse and General Shoop, but the boys have generously left the responsibility for financing as well as the starring role to me. In the early part of the script my entire time was taken up with finding out about another me—me, the husband and father—and for a few years while the picture business was in a gentle slump, I was so busy trying to be made of money that I had no time to care whether I was already made of protein or not.

Then once again the scene changed, a well established character re-entered, and a new act began. Again I was in Chicago, this time on my way to New York to do *Faithfully Yours* with Ann Southern, my first Broadway play in fifteen years. I decided to stop en route, visit Gene Feuchtinger and take a few brush-up lessons at the Perfect Voice Institute. And I am sure that second meeting will add many happy years to my life, for Gene did more than help me with my voice. He rekindled my interest in nutrition.

When I dropped in on Gene I was definitely in that condition we have described as *over-fed and under-nourished* (maybe even a little hollow). I had forgotten what it was like to feel *really* good—the absence of actual pain had become my barometer—and I was complacently accepting as normal that "tired-run-down-feeling," the feeling of not being up to "par." Truthfully, like many people in early and middle life, I had lost the idea of what "par" should or could be. I certainly wasn't sick—but I was far from well. I was having trouble with persistent colds. I was over-weight. I was tired. To all of which Dr. Feuchtinger said something old and familiar: "You sound to me like you are not getting the right things to eat."

Now he didn't prescribe any immediate corrective diet for a busy and headstrong actor-husband-father who had come quite simply for a few singing lessons. But he fanned the flame of my rekindled interest by sending me away with some books. I began to read, to study with an open mind to see whether this matter of nutrition deserved some more serious adventuring.

And I came to believe that it did.

I came to believe that Methuselah and those giants were

not mere legend, nor characters from antiquity whose achievements could be explained away on the grounds that they *counted* differently in those days—say a month for a year or some such. The facts seemed to indicate that they *lived* and *ate* differently, that those people were living off food just as God prepared it for them, growing in rich, fertile soil from which the plants extracted and transformed the natural riches to become the sustenance of man, again according to a plan God prepared. They ate fish. They ate meat, but there were many things they did not eat and many so-called refinements developed by civilization of which they never heard. Their instincts were primitive—more like the Eskimos and the Masai warriors—but I was convinced they had produced results.

Now as I read, studied, and experimented I was plowing deep the shallow half-knowledge which had once led me to accept fadism. I was learning a lot, trying this, trying that, and gradually I evolved some simple, sensible rules for sound eating, rules as old as Methuselah and as new as the science of bio-chemistry. These I want to share with you. They worked!

The *proof* was in the eating. As I learned what good nutrition was my vitality picked up, my weight reduced, and physically I knew what it was *really* like to feel well. Whoever said *"you are what you eat"* was right. My dad was right when he said "you are protein." I was protein. Of course, as I've hinted, in my experience they were only *one-third right for those who wish to be truly at the top of their form*. But it is where I began, and so I'll try to follow the directions the King gave the White Rabbit in Alice's Wonderland, to "begin at the beginning, and go on till you come to the end: then stop." In that way the other two-thirds will unfold before we are finished, to show exactly how I believe we can be whole, wholesome, vital beings—Man-As-Man-Should-Be (also Woman), starting right now!

Chapter 5

The Mystery and Miracle of You

We are repeatedly informed that we live in an age of miracles, yet to me the greatest miracle of any age is *us* —you, me, the guy next door, my smallest daughter, a Masai warrior—that amazing entity known as Man, wherever and however you find him. We are all Life itself manifesting from the invisible to the visible at the highest level we know —growing, unfolding, thinking, creating, re-creating, working, playing; and since life is the prime mystery of our planet, we, you and I, are both *mystery* and *miracle*.

If you don't believe that, consider for a moment that body you're running around in!

Floyd Parsons once said: "Engineers are prone to talk of the efficiency of modern machines. But no machine is as efficient as man himself. Where can we find a pump as perfect as the human heart? If we treat it right it stays on the job for more than 600,000 hours, making 4,320 strokes and pumping fifteen gallons an hour.

"We have no telegraphic mechanism equal to our nervous system; no radio so efficient as the voice and ear; no camera as perfect as the human eye; no ventilating plant as wonderful as the nose, lungs, and skin. No electrical switchboard can compare with the spinal cord."

And what, in my eyes, raises this efficiency to miracle level is that all these functions, plus a thousand more, are carried on without our conscious effort or knowledge, at a rate of speed and with an automatic intelligence almost incredible to us, though we live with them, on them, and by them. It's more complicated than a thousand IBM machines.

To me this body is more like a giant factory or a great scientific laboratory than a machine, a laboratory where millions of cells form, function, die, and are replaced; where food is digested and assimilated, transformed by body chemistry, rushed through the blood stream to vital spots where special glands mastermind the manufacture of mighty midgets called hormones, launching them directly into the blood, and other mighty midgets called enzymes go about their fantastic function of breaking up our food as it passes along the digestive tract and helping to absorb it. And all this, day and night, without our conscious volition!

I consciously lift my hands, move my arms, open my mouth, sing, run, drive a car, fly my plane, but who tells my heart to beat? Who tells my eyes to focus, to blink? I couldn't learn enough in a thousand years to direct the fascinating, precise, myriad operations that take place in my body during one hour. Napoleon himself was never a sufficiently informed general to plan the amazing warfare waged by the white corpuscles in his body at the slightest sign of infection. If I were left on my own to order these functions for five short minutes—well, goodbye, Bob!

I must just accept the miracle, and thank God.

But, as Floyd Parsons points out, such a mechanism is worthy of the highest respect and care, although he believes it seldom gets it, "and that is why," he concludes, "the sales of medical services, whether in operations or convalescence, hospital or home, is measured in billions of dollars."

Now the question arises—at least it did with me—what constitutes the highest respect and care? Since unconscious intelligence or instinct directs this super-complicated laboratory, shouldn't we have a built-in instinct for its care? If not, how did man progress down these thousands of years before the science of medicine, nutrition, and bio-chemistry made his functions and his needs less of a mystery if not less of a miracle?

Education vs. Instinct

It's my firm belief that man not only *should* have such instincts but that he *did* have them. Methuselah had them. Noah had them. Moses had them. It was being Good Animals which laid the foundation for being Giants among men, and animals retain those built-in instincts today. The animal, in his wild state, doesn't need to study the body or a book or be educated to his needs. He instinctively selects what is good for him—rejects what is not. A lion doesn't need to learn about protein to know that he's a meat-eater, any more than a squirrel has to be spanked for killing chickens and coaxed to eat nuts. It takes a good deal of ingenuity to get a wild animal to do or take what isn't good for him—even a meat-eating domesticated poodle won't develop a taste for *bon-bons* and *antipasto* without putting up more-than-human resistance.

The wild animal rarely gets too fat or too thin. He usually keeps his vitality, hair, teeth, and alert senses for his allotted span unless maimed or killed by accident, avalanche, landslide, famine, drought—some event which has nothing to do with the state of his health. The same, as we have pointed out, holds true of the Masai warrior, the Eskimo who has not as yet met "civilization," the jungle Indians of the Amazon. Yet these men, like the wild animals, have never heard of nutrition, bio-chemistry, balanced diet, and the like.

Why is it, then, that you and I are in such need of these sciences? Why is it suddenly necessary for man to pick apart the lovely miracle of the body and see what makes it tick? Be "educated" as to what is good for him and what is not?

The answer seems to be that, over years and years of civilizing man to artificial ways of living and eating, he has lost his natural instinct. Over-civilized man has ceased to be a Good Animal. His instincts can't be trusted.

This didn't happen yesterday. Nor even the day before. By the time Moses, his own natural force unabated, led his captive people out of highly civilized Egypt, he felt he had to give them health laws as well as spiritual laws for their over-all well-being. Nor is this opinion either thoroughly modern nor exclusively my own. Benjamin Franklin, when he and our other fore-fathers were nursing our country in its cradle, observed: "In general, mankind, since the improvement of cookery, eats twice as much as nature requires." At another time he said: "I saw few men die of hunger, of eating—a hundred thousand."

If man has lost his God-given instinct to know what to eat, how much to eat, and when to eat, then this must be replaced by a *conscious understanding of our miracle-laboratory—the body—its functions and requirements;* and we must be educated to give it consciously that "highest respect and care" by providing for it the *materials* and *conditions* necessary not only to keep it from breaking down (being ill), but functioning at top form at all ages.

I have just re-read the above paragraph and if it doesn't scare you, it scares me. The tone is about the same as the opening of a profound lecture I heard in the early days of my interest in nutrition—and the lecturer proceeded in the same vein. Afterwards I overheard three men seated in front of me comment.

"I tell you," said one enthusiastically, "this speaker dives deeper into the truth than any other I ever heard."

"Yes," agreed the second man, "and he can stay down longer."

"Yes," said the third, "and come up drier!"

Now, I have every intention of diving into the truth, as I understand it, but I have no intention of diving very deep or staying down very long. In trying to understand the body's *functions* and *requirements* I don't mean to give a casual medical study nor a superficial, accordion-pleated view of physiology. I'm not qualified to offer the long or short course in either. Besides, it isn't necessary to dive that deep. All that is necessary for our purposes is to show *why* we need to provide our body-laboratory with certain specific materials (it's the real reason that we eat at all, regardless of what our stomach or palate claims), where these materials can be obtained (the importance of selecting what we eat), what happens when there's a shortage (later we will discuss some easy ways to recognize the common deficiency symptoms—in relation to youthfulness and vitality, as well as beauty), and some sensible rules for correcting shortages and maintaining the daily flow of materials needed to keep our laboratory fully efficient at all times and ages.

It's all very simple. It's all very logical. Nature usually is—and remember, these are nature's laws, not mine. The whole idea is to educate ourselves back to where we departed from nature's instinct. I have adopted for myself seven general rules for getting the needed materials under normal circumstances and seven more for maintaining proper conditions. These, when you *read* them in the following chapters, add up to a fourteen-point program—but actually, if you *live* them and don't stop with reading, they add up to more vigor, more vitality, more sparkle than you have ever known.

In later chapters we'll deal more specifically with recognizing and correcting undesirable conditions—beauty problems, figure problems, even personality flaws—as well as the individual temptations and pitfalls that must be watched at various ages—in the teens—as young adults—during middle life—as senior citizens. But here's a word of warning. I don't want any dissatisfied readers. I have no sure-nutritional-cure for corns, a moulting appendix, or the like. I'm not trying to take over for the physician or the specialist trained in nutrition or bio-chemistry. I'm no more qualified to diagnose or prescribe in the case of illness than I am to rewrite Shakespeare. If you have a specialized health problem, by all means consult a specialist.

Any other course is fadism or foolishness.

In this book we are going to deal generally with things I know about. I am highly qualified to tell you what has helped me—and I can vouch for the fact that every science, medical or academic, which has your personal well-being as its goal, endorses the premise that sound nutrition is the foundation of a sound body, that it can both help to prevent and correct deficiency diseases, that it is of real importance in transforming that tired, run-down you into You-As-You-Should-Be.

I Promise You.

The specialists have written many fine books and papers. I have drawn liberally upon their years of research and experiments in formulating my own program—for theirs is not a secret knowledge but a knowledge they are dedicated to trying to pass along to you and me. Later we'll take a quick look at some of the responsible work by foundations and individuals being done today to advance our understanding. In diving very deep into the wonderful world of nutrition I have never come up dry, and I don't think you would. But I'm not for turning a guy loose with an aqua-lung before he has learned to swim. Unless you have first been introduced to fundamentals I think you only become hopelessly confused and unnecessarily bewildered if plunged in over your head.

I remember that I, personally, with the great enthusiasm of the beginner, dived early with the experts, went down two hundred feet the first time, and came up puzzled and discouraged. "How can I remember all this?" I demanded of anyone who would listen. "It's too complicated. It's a whole new way of life. I'm a struggling actor. I haven't the time. I haven't the money."

But now, here we are, me talking to you, a layman talking to a layman, and I will honestly confess that all I really lacked was the patience to simplify and adapt what I read, and the will power to make a decision to *live* it. If, in this book, I err according to expert opinions a little on the side of over-simplification, it has its advantages. We want to start with a basic program *you can understand right now, put into practice right now, and from which you can get results starting, say, tomorrow morning.*

If charts and gory details are omitted, it is not an oversight. I may appear to be a gay deceiver (that's just one of my various screen roles). Actually I'm a deliberate, thoughtful guy. Just ask my Mary! And I figure the charts and the·delightful diagrams of what lies between our skeletons and our skins have been most thoroughly done in other places. There's a bibliography in the back of this book and any of you who are interested can dive into that up to fifty fathoms —once you're used to the water.

My aim is to help you get your feet wet, to help you learn to swim. I don't want to make anybody an expert. I just want to show you the best way I've found to be a thoroughly happy guy—or gal.

I hope I can make you wake up and do something about your health. Think! Be aware!

I want you to be hep—not hipped—nutrition-wise.

Now I don't say you won't want to change friends and influence strangers once you've caught on. That's inevitable. Look at me—writing a book yet. And I'm still conspicuously alert at parties. You'll notice me circulating happily— "What? You're nervous? Irritable? Did you ever try a lullaby diet?" (page 153) "No pep, pal? You fold on the set every afternoon at three? Why not try some lime in your

drinking water?" (page 153) "Bloodshot eyes that feel like
there's sand in 'em? Those great big beautiful eyes? Maybe
you need vitamin B$_2$. (page 69).

You'll be doing that routine, too. That's the mark of the
enthusiast, someone for whom this program has worked. But
the expert is something else again.

I remember standing next to two distinguished guests at
a large Hollywood party one night. One was a leading New
York stage actress, the other a famous London surgeon.
Neither seemed interested in participating as the party, a
movie-land command performance for most of us, flowed
noisily around them. Finally the man from Harley Street,
courteously trying to make conversation, said, "I am always
a little lost at these big gatherings."

"I used to be," purred the actress. "But not since I've
taken up Italian and French. Now I stand here and practice
my languages. I translate everything the men say into Italian
and everything the women say into French."

The surgeon's eyes gleamed as he surveyed the glittering
assembly. "And I," he said happily, "I mentally diagnose
and dissect the blighters."

Somehow this made a deep, if shuddery impression on me.
And while I know you will have such immediate success with
the way of life outlined here that you will feel irrepressibly
compelled to share your discoveries, I should hate to be
responsible for focusing your mind on the body in such technical detail that you might cease to see people and see instead
perambulating laboratories containing so many miles of
upper and lower colon, of blood vessels and arteries, so many
hardworking pulsating cells all deceptively packaged to look
like Deborah Kerr, maybe. It's much nicer to see Deborah
Kerr.

So depend on it—any omissions are deliberate and pur-
poseful, but in no way detrimental to the effectiveness of the
rules.

Here is what I promise you about the simple program that follows:

It has helped me—it can help you.

It has changed my life—it can change yours.

If I can remember and apply it—so can you.

If I have time to follow it—you do too.

If I could afford it when I started it—you can afford it as well.

And now—let's dive in.

Chapter 6

You Are What You Eat

Do you remember the old game called Three Kingdoms? Well, it's enjoying a revival at our dinner table. Melinda, our number one daughter, looking at the flowers in the center of the table announces: "I'm vegetable," and we ply her with questions until we guess correctly that she is the lowest sweet pea on the south side of the floral piece. Patricia, number two daughter, is "mineral" and it's fairly easy to figure out that she's mommy's wedding ring. But the other night, very small Tony, number two son, came up with a stumper: "I'm Bob Cummings," he said, "what am I?"

It's a good question. Answers vary depending on whose angle you take. To me, and to a minister friend of mine, I'd say I am mind, body and spirit. I know some critics who'd say I'm mostly animal (say "Ham!"). In the laboratory I'd analyze as human animal (Good Animal, I trust), but at the dinner table, when the offspring watch me eat, it would appear that it requires all Three Kingdoms to keep one Good Animal functioning.

Animal, Vegetable, and Mineral

The foods we eat, the fluids we drink, the air we breathe must supply all the essential raw materials our cells need for growth, repair, and energy if we are to be healthy, vital, energetic, and look and act our age properly. (Why not sweet sixty as well as sweet sixteen?) Specifically, we eat to provide energy, plus replacement and repair materials—and we reach out to all Three Kingdoms, animal, vegetable, and mineral, to get our supplies.

There's an ominous if lush cliché that reminds one of Persian dancing girls, or Roman couches in the days of Nero, or soldiers going off to battle, which goes: "Eat, drink, and be merry, for tomorrow we die." Modern nutritionists could brush it up a bit and make it currently accurate. "Eat and drink incorrectly and tomorrow you'll be a sight deader than you ought to be," or "Eat and drink correctly and tomorrow you'll be merry."

To eat correctly is the beginning of wisdom so far as giving our fantastic, obliging body proper respect and care is concerned—and the beginning of the beginning lies in that one word—*Protein*. Protein comes from the Greek word meaning "to come first" and that's exactly where it belongs nutrition-wise. Now there *are* other foods, some of them vital—vitamins, minerals, etc.—and we'll deal with them shortly. But protein is Number One.

Scientifically its importance was stated this way by Dr. William Albrecht: "Life is not passed from one fat globule to another, nor from one grain of starch to another, but only from one protein to another protein molecule."

Unscientifically stated by me it sounds like this: "No protein—no life." How basic can a thing be? Can anything in the material world be much more important than that?

I remember some lines in an old patter routine I did years ago where the judge says, "Why did you steal the $75,000?"

And the defendant says, "I was hungry." How hungry can you get? It sounds ridiculous. But, if you really understand protein-hunger you can get hungry $75,000 worth. Or much, much more, depending on the price you place on the vitality and energy you need to do your job (to earn!) and enjoy the world. You could even say depending on the price or value you put on your life.

Do you find that hard to believe? So I'll explain—but first let me say that this is the "think" chapter, the answer to why we need to provide our body-laboratory with certain specific material. We're going to investigate the theory behind all this. The next chapters are the "do" chapters but I've found that unconvinced people simply read a while, admire, smile and say, "isn't that interesting" and the next time they hear the word *protein* they decide it's something the Russians invented to spread on a Sputnik. However, if you find yourself wanting more details so you can start practicing what I preach, you only have a short wait.

Proteins at Work

In the matter of life and death here is a case reported by Dr. Weston A. Price,* in which a minister brought to him an undersized, suffering little boy who appeared to be dying.

Johnny's body was emaciated, racked by deep coughing. For eight months he had had convulsions of increasing severity and during one of them, nearly two months earlier, he had fractured his leg. It was still in a cast, still unhealed. The minister had heard that Dr. Price was doing marvelous things in restoring health through nutrition and he asked him to help the tragic little fellow. Dr. Price made up a high-protein gruel to which he added some highly nutritious butter oil he had developed, and spooned it slowly to the motionless boy.

---

* *Nutrition and Physical Degeneration,* by Weston A. Price. The American Academy of Applied Nutrition, Los Angeles, California, 1939.

The boy slept—without the aid of barbiturates. The following day he had five servings of the porridge. His mother continued to feed it to him for four weeks. His leg healed. The convulsions ceased. He gained weight and began to grow. At the end of another six weeks he was harassing his mother with all the normal, welcome mischief of the whole, high-spirited youngster God meant him to be.

A miracle?

Perhaps. A miracle of nutrition. The miracle, according to Dr. Price, of supplying his body with its prime building material—protein. Johnny, Dr. Price felt, certainly without his mother's knowledge, certainly without her conscious consent, had been dying of protein-hunger.

That is the story of a child and a tragic ignorance. Here is a reverse case history, that of a handsome, healthy man, a dedicated, informed nutritionist who was leading an energetic, happy, satisfying life and decided, for his own verification and personal experience, to test the results of protein deficiency in his own body. Lelord Kordel,* over a period of eight months gradually cut his daily protein intake to a point he knew to be inadequate. After several months he found that writing or lecturing at night left him "head-and-body-weary." Then he began to feel fatigue from his accustomed daily routine. At night he didn't want to do anything but sit in his chair in a sort of exhausted stupor. His good appetite flagged and so did his normal pleasure in people and events. He found himself irritable, "too tired" to play with his two small sons. Sounds like that "old tired feeling," no? In his own words he reports: "I was not the man I used to be. If I had not been aware of the cause for my 'slipping,' I would have been panicked by the unpleasant discovery which most of you have already faced: *I was losing my grip.*"

How? Because he had suddenly gotten old? No. By de-

---

* *Eat and Grow Younger,* by Lelord Kordel. The World Publishing Co., New York, 1952.

priving his body of its ace building material. And who knows what would have happened next? Because Mr. Kordel had *gone as far as he cared to go*. He knew how to put a stop to this—and he did it. When you have finished reading this you will know how—and the rest is up to you.

Malnutrition is a little like a street car starting off in the very best part of town and bound for Skid Row. Once you have found where this trolley takes you, you can get off at any stop—and by following the rules, take the next trolley back. The length of time it takes to get back where you started from depends on how soon you change your direction. And the biggest coin you possess for that return fare is *protein*.

Just what does this master food do?

First, protein is the basic body building material.

From the delicate brain tissues to those thousands of miles of blood vessels we weren't going to talk about, your blood plasma, red blood cells, those magic hormones and enzymes, muscles, bone, every cell in your body needs protein for growth and maintenance. Except for bile and urine that whole fascinating façade you present to the world is composed of protein in some form.

Protein Is Replacement Material

The body is constantly changing, renewing, assimilating, eliminating, discarding the old and reaching for the new. Internal and external secretions (such as digestive juices, enzymes, hormones, tears, skin oil) must be produced without a let up if we are to function constantly at top form. There must be new red blood cells to replace the defunct ones. White blood cells, intestinal cells, and the like are in need of replacement. The cells of our skin, hair, nails, are destroyed and new ones needed. Your body is *living,* circulating, regenerating, constantly. Unlike the fuel you put in your automobile, the fuel you give your body actually becomes a part of you, and the used parts are then sloughed off. Each food trip brings in new supplies. The cells release used-up protein and reach out for more. If you haven't supplied enough to go around a shortage appears somewhere and at that somewhere a deficiency occurs. Some part or parts of your body is starved for protein.

Protein Is Repair and Defense Material

Nature has designed antibodies as our defenders against the bacteria, virus, and so forth which constantly attack our well being. *Nature provided us with immunities that can come to us in food.* These antibodies are formed of protein. Scientists have shown by experiment that a hundred times more of these vital security guards appear in the bloodstream when our diets are high in protein.

Does all this convince you? Are you now a True Believer? Because there's more—much more.

Without protein youngsters won't grow, between-agers droop, and oldsters don't mend, among other facts. Vitality is low, tissues shrivel (horrible thought!), broken bones don't mend normally. Dental cavities appear, sparkling eyes dim and seeing eyes deceive (there IS a difference between "c" and "o," between "P" and "F" on the eye chart) digestion falters (did you ever rumble in a complete silence?) and silhouettes are distorted (*all* in the wrong places). And then there are those mighty midgets—*enzymes*. Enzymes are the agents that do the greatest part of our digestive work and enzymes—so far as science has been able to analyze them —are made of protein.

We have already mentioned those Master Minds, the endocrine glands and their offspring, the hormones. We'll mention them in more detail later in their starring role but right here we'll put in a Coming Attraction with them taking second billing to Pal Protein. Protein could be said to be the Angel behind every body drama—the butter-and-egg man, the Money bags, the *backer* because without this backing—no stars, no script, no direction, *no show*. For our coming attraction on the Glands that direct the Hormones to go out and stimulate our organs into giving a top performance, to make sure your actions and reactions are dynamic, your health radiant, your good looks fadeless, that you keep your vitality regardless of calendar age, it is enough to say here that *both the glands and hormones are basically protein.*

Make up your mind to feed your glands *right now,* and *right now* you have made a decision that will change your life. It will put your show on the road. It will give you a hit instead of a miss.

Now can you see why $75,000 would be a small price to place on protein hunger?

But here's happy news. You won't have to steal a penny. *Good nutrition is not a matter of money* as is evidenced by the fact that, if you are a parrot owner, pretty Polly probably is better fed, protein-wise, than you are, and that on sunflower seeds. Now, as the Ring-leader in the circus says when the lights dim on the center arena, "May I call your attention to the ring on our right. The new stars you are about to observe are of small size but great magnitude. May I introduce to you the . . ."

Vitamin Family

There was a cartoon in the New Yorker some time ago showing a prisoner being given the third degree and the caption under it read: "I don't know what made me do it —some sort of vitamin deficiency maybe."

But this may not be such a joke after all. Many authorities are coming to believe that malnutrition is not only crippling to the body, but crippling to the mind. Karl B. Mickey* puts

* *Man and the Soil*, Karl B. Mickey, Chicago, International Harvester Co., 1945.

it thus: "Where physical stamina is lacking the will lacks power; and the process of thinking . . . is profoundly influenced by the state of general health." Prominent researchers, among them Weston A. Price, Alexis Carrel, and Ernest A. Hooton—have attributed a percentage of juvenile delinquency as well as adult insanity and criminality to the moral consequences of physical degeneration—and many leaders agree that the degenerative diseases have their roots mostly in accumulated nutritional deficiencies.

Very big thoughts, those, for very big deficiencies—and here we have been discussing youth, beauty, and vitality! We're about to get back to them, too, but before we do, and to short circuit putting vitamins in a bad light, let's face another fascinating trick nature has concocted for us. She has so designed our body and its needs that, while the material of which we need the *most* is protein, we find it isn't the *only* one, and that it can't work alone. No protein can do all a good little protein should without the cooperating presence of vitamins and minerals. Dr. Charles E. Dutchess, medical director of an Eastern research laboratory, feels the public needs to know the necessity of eating "plenty of lean meat, eggs, milk (our friend protein in his market state), vitamins and minerals obtained from a broad selection of meats, fruits, and vegetables."

It is interesting to watch the interdependence of this trio as our nutrition script unfolds. Meanwhile, back to the Vitamin Story.

One nutritionist, when asked to define these dietary assets, said, "About the best definition we can give is—*vitamins are the substances that make us ill if we don't eat them.*"

They were noted, if not named, by Christopher Columbus in the early fifteen hundreds on one of his voyages to the New World. Several of his sailors became ill with scurvy, a disease rightfully dreaded by seamen since whole crews died of it. When Columbus sighted an island the suffering men begged to be put ashore to die in peace. The ships landed them and sailed on. Some months later, on the return voyage, they again passed within sight of the island and were amazed to see men standing on the shore waving to them. Once again they landed, this time to find the dying men fully recovered. Because of this miraculous cure Columbus named the island Curaçao, or "cure" in Portuguese.

Years later the miracle was explained when a ship's "surgeon" performed a simple experiment. Once again the crew was down with scurvy but this time the doctor, Dr. Lind, ordered that half of them be kept on the regular fare of salt pork and sea biscuits while to the diet of the other men he added lime juice. Those getting the lime juice recovered—as had the sailors with Columbus when they got fresh fruit on the "miracle" island—and when Dr. Lind added the fresh juice to the diet of the other half of the crew, they, too, threw off the symptoms of scurvy. From this came the custom of feeding lime juice daily to British sailors (and from it, too, came their nickname "limeys"). Later on this miracle "substance" in the limes "that made them sick if they didn't eat it" was named Vitamin C. Beri-beri, the disease which translated, means "I can't" and which kills millions annually in the Far East, begins as a slow loss of energy and movement and ends in death. It, too, proved to be a deficiency, this time of Vitamin B_1.

Now this is very dramatic but you and I are not fighting a personal battle with scurvy or beri-beri—nor are we likely to. But here are a few common instances where vitamin lacks can show up at home. Poor growth, heart disturbances, infection, pyorrhea, nervousness, muscular inflammation described by us over the back fence as "lumbago," or "bursitis," or "rheumatism," (depending on the location of the ache), respiratory infections (among them that Common Cold), skin problems including undue oiliness or undue dryness, lack of pep, night blindness (pilots know best!) can be connected with not eating those little substances.

Here are some other interesting facts about the vitamin

family. Whereas we need a great deal of protein, the body requires only small amounts of each vitamin—but in the delicate scale of our laboratory, these amounts can tip the scales from disease to health, even from death to life.

Now here is how important their supporting role is—*proteins and vitamins work together*. Those enzymes that do our digestive work are, as we have said, protein. Certain of these protein enzymes actually take part in your body's use of vitamins and the compliment is returned because certain vitamins affect the body's production of protein enzymes. Also, vitamins and those wondrous hormones are interdependent. In other words, you can't expect proteins to function properly without vitamins—and vitamins can't do their job without protein. And now let's add to these the third member of the trio mentioned by Dr. Dutchess. . . .

Minerals

It's tantalizing to think that over thirteen members of the mineral kingdom are vitally necessary to our body-laboratory. Fortunately, the more expensive ones are not required and we can actually save on having to buy gold and silver for holes in our teeth by getting some of the less costly minerals into our stomach. Fortunately again, nature doesn't require us to mine our minerals but has arranged for the animal and vegetable kingdom to do the digging for us—fish, among other foods, providing us with iodine, and oysters and figs being excellent copper collectors.

But even when the amounts needed are very small the part they play in our well-being is very large.

In a published report to the New York State Joint Legislative Committee on Nutrition (1947) Dr. C. Ward Crampton stated that the American diet was more deficient in *calcium* than in any other single food element. Calcium has been more highly publicized than most minerals as necessary for building bones and teeth—so we concentrate on giving it to babies, children with leg cramps or "growing pains," pregnant women, and nursing mothers. But Dr. Crampton points out that—*"calcium poverty is one common cause of aging that can be corrected."*

Since our nerves, heart, teeth, brain cells and blood all demand calcium, if we send down an insufficient supply a very hot argument ensues as to who gets the available material with the blood usually carrying away the laurels (or calcium). Mineral deficiencies accumulate—and shortly the bones become fragile, fracture easily, teeth decay, heart muscles and brain cells don't do all that's expected of them —not because they are "aging," but because they are "starving."

Mineral deficiencies, as with the other members of the trio, show up in personality flaws as well as physical difficulties. Calcium affords a good example of this. It is common knowledge that an iron deficiency in the blood can make us anemic, or at least wan and pale. But without calcium in solution in the blood we can have a real personality change —the nerves don't send out proper messages—we are irritable and nervous—we might even develop an impossible amount of temperament. (You can see where a temptation arises when I am on the set somewhere with an overly temperamental star—and I think "the poor thing may not be so very long on talent as so very short on calcium.")

You probably know that you need calcium for hair and fingernails, but did you know that, if they are dull, fading, and breaking, you may lack *sulphur?* Did you know that sulphur is vital to skin beauty? That lack of *iodine* may be responsible for your silhouette problem (pudgy or scrawny or just out of balance—the details to be found in Chapter 17? Are you exhausted by the heat? Enervated, dull, when the mercury climbs? Well, *salt* occurs in solution in all your body fluids and the protoplasms of your cells. On a hot day or in a hot spot (factory, movie set, baking oven, or party where you show up in costume of Eve to find that everyone else is in full evening dress) you lose a lot of water in genteel perspiration. And with the water, you lose salt—and a salt shortage results in heat exhaustion. Do you find the opposite sex losing their appeal? Do you find yourself losing your appeal for them? A diminishing of your sex powers, your physical attraction and virility? Well, your sex glands, in addition to protein foods and vitamins, need *iron* and *copper*.

Once again we find that this trio, composed of protein, vitamins, minerals, is not just a pick-up of separate vocalists who sing together because they like the sound, but comprises an inseparable instrument, like the strings, bow, and case of a violin—one will make no music at all without the other.

A National Academy of Science research team has emphasized that the minerals, *potassium, phosphorus,* and *magnesium,* are essential in the diet for all body-building protein foods. We find calcium and phosphorus needed for bones, but vitamin "D" controls the retention, absorption, and distribution of these minerals to the bone. We know the endocrine glands and their hormones are basically protein, that hormones and vitamins are interdependent, and now we find that neither of them will function, separately or together, except in the presence of certain minerals.

If this all sounds almost as complicated as it does fascinating—well, it is. But it's necessary to get a little complicated before we can get simple. And we're not through yet. Dramatically speaking, our nutrition script is a bomb. It reminds me of a big-time Hollywood producer I knew who was giving his script-writers a pep talk. He was the sort of fellow who wanted every picture super-colossal and he was ordering them to deliver.

"Got any suggestions?" one writer asked.

"Sure," said the producer, shifting his cigar. "Start with an earthquake—then work up to a climax."

The Energy Twins

If you have really accepted what we've discussed so far about proteins, vitamins, and minerals and *are prepared to do something about it,* you've just been through a nutritional earthquake that's going to shake up your whole life. We've spotlighted a trio of building materials, proteins, vitamins, minerals, of which the average American diet contains *far too little,* or none at all. Now, for a climax, we come to the energy twins, *carbohydrates* and *fats,* of which we are probably getting *far too much, the wrong kinds, and in the wrong combinations.*

Here the calorie counters, some thirty-five-million Americans who are all fussed up about being overweight, come into their own territory. But simply counting calories, while it undoubtedly slices pounds, is *not* the most effective way to be slim and *vital.* Girth control, like every other phase of bodily health, starts with a proper understanding of nutrition—and so we will take a close look at the energy twins as they affect our daily diet.

We have agreed that we eat to provide the body with *building* and *repair* material and to produce *energy* for our cells to do their work and keep the body warm. (And this, although it may horrify the gourmet or the member of the Cordon Bleu, was nature's single original idea!) The units of food energy released by your food are counted in *calories.* Carbohydrates (the technical name under which starches and sugars travel) and fats are high in calories. They are energy foods, as is also protein. When we eat, the digestive processes convert the foods to glucose (a particular kind of animal sugar) which is carried about and distributed by the blood stream. Blood sugar is as important to life as the air we breathe—it is the sugar which burns in the oxygen we breathe, and is the energy fuel of every cell of the body. What we eat is converted at the rate of one hundred percent of the carbohydrates, fifty-six percent of the proteins, and ten percent of the fats.

Obviously, unless their use is misunderstood or abused, carbohydrates have a place in our diet or nature would not have provided them so lavishly. But here's the rub. Nature has provided carbohydrates in such abundance in natural foods that it is almost impossible *not* to get enough of them. We do not have to reach out for starch and sugar since every plant, both fruit and vegetable, is a little carbohydrate factory of nature's own design. If we concentrate on a high protein diet together with the foods that provide the best sources of vitamins and minerals, we will get our carbohydrates in the exact form that nature intended we should. These are the *right kind* of sugars and starches and we will *not* have to count calories.

If, however, we add *empty calories* to our diet at mealtime, foods containing starch and sugar unmixed with the vital building materials, we run two risks, very grave ones. First, we will take on more fuel than we can burn up . . . and the excess will be stored in embarrassing places, putting a great strain on the organs of the body as well as the eye of the beholder. (I can't resist the gory detail that it takes yards and yards of blood vessels to support one extra pound of fat.)

Second, it will satisfy our *appetite* but not our *hunger*. It just hides the hunger. Your appetite is your instinctive body cry for nourishment—and if you send down a load of carbohydrates (starch or sugar) unmixed with building materials (no proteins, minerals, vitamins) you are sending a load of empty cars into a famine area. There is much commotion at the station when the train arrives and the appetite, thinking it has done its job, goes to rest. But the hidden hunger goes on for the cars carry nothing but calories, and while you may get a momentary lift from the "quick energy" you'll be in worse shape when that passes because you are that much further behind in building materials, the deficiencies are accumulating, and the only reserves on hand are an over-abundance of heating fuel to be stored somewhere.

Here we have the case of the individual who is overweight, but under-fed—(who is "hollow"), or over-fed (on starch and sugar) but under-nourished (by a lack of protein, minerals and vitamins).

It just doesn't make sense, does it?

A New York physician who specialized in reducing put this quaint sign in his waiting room:

> If your coat is no longer button-y,
> Ask yourself: Is it gluttony?

A glutton he described as "the guy who takes the piece of French pastry you wanted." Translated, that means the guy who wants all the unnatural sugar and starch that your civilized taste thinks it wants, too. But nature didn't plan it that way. Did you ever hear of a pair of tigers in the jungle fighting over a chocolate eclair? Or a deer headed for a field of spring grass who could be lured by a pan of fudge?

Here's the key to proper carbohydrates without counting calories and taking a chance that even those few you send down will be empty. Good carbohydrates are always in a train load of good building material. Natural fruits, vegetables, even meats, natural sources of protein, vitamins, and minerals, will give you your sugars and starches in the right form and proper amounts.

Fats are composed of glycerin and fatty "acids." These, one of our most concentrated forms of energy, are also almost always found in nature in combination either with protein or carbohydrates—and let's say right here that *small amounts of fats* are a prime building material as well as source of energy. You'll never have that vital health, those calm nerves, that skin-I'd-love-to-touch on a fat-free diet. Once again we note the interdependence nature specializes in. Fats work with our other building materials to give full performance, combining with the mineral phosphorus to form part of every cell, particularly in brain and nerve tissues. Fats burn best in the presence of carbohydrates and some of the vitamin family are fat-soluble and fats are necessary to help us absorb them. Nature has given us a thin layer of fat just under the skin to act as insulator against sudden temperature changes, as a protection for muscles and nerves, and thus emaciated or too thin people "wear their nerves on the outside," are restless and irritable.

You can see now the reason for the statement—"you are what you eat." Your body is in constant need of proteins, vitamins, minerals, carbohydrates, and fats—and these we get from the Three Kingdoms—Animal, Vegetable, Mineral. Here we have tried to show logically *what materials* this miracle-body of ours requires, and *why* the materials are needed in order to give it the "high respect and care" it must have if it is to live up to our demands on it—our demands that it stay young, vital, well, attractive. Now we will proceed to *where* we get these vital materials and *how*, under what conditions, they will do the most for us.

"Seven Rules for Flying High"

Irvin S. Cobb, a great American humorist, used to tell about walking along a road in Georgia after a giant rainstorm and coming upon Henry sitting in an easy chair by the kitchen door, fishing in a puddle of water.

"Henry, you old fool," said Cobb, "what are you doing there?"

"Boss," said Henry, "I'se just fishin' a little."

"Don't you know there's no fish there?" asked Cobb.

"Yes, suh," said Henry. "I know dat, but dis yer place is so handy."

Henry and you and I have something in common. When it comes to nutrition most of us, even when we know better, even when we realize we've been fishin' in an empty puddle and failing our bodies *before* they fail us, even after promising ourselves we'll do something about it, wind up sittin' in the same old kitchen fishin' out of the same old diet because the old way "is so handy."

The hold of habit is strong. It takes an effort to change it. The most important step you're going to have to take if you mean to experience any improvement is to *make up your mind that you are going to give these rules a try.*

Here, in brief, are the seven general rules I have adopted
for getting the needed materials under normal circumstances.

One: *Get Enough and More Than Enough Protein Daily.*
Two: *Vitamins Daily for Vigor and Vitality.*
Three: *Daily Minerals Are a Must.*
Four: *Handle Carbohydrates with Care.*
Five: *Fats Are Food and We Need a Limited Amount of
           Certain Fats Every Day.*
Six: *Fluids Are Fundamental. . . . Six to Ten Glasses of
           Liquid Every Twenty-four Hours.*
Seven: *Plan, Market and Cook with an Open Eye on Health,
           Beauty and Zest.*

In the next few chapters we will deal in detail with "where
the body materials we require can be obtained" and "how to
maintain a daily flow of supply." I worked these out for my
personal use. They did the trick for me. But their soundness
is also indicated by published experiments in the scientific
field.

Remember, *good* nutrition is not *fad* nutrition and I've
tried to stay with established concepts. Fads can be fun, can
capture the imagination, promise a lot, but they can also be
unbalanced and even dangerous. I have tried to avoid them
too because they overlook the *unity of nutrition.* The body
is a unity—even though in words it must unfold as a series
of separate parts and activities—and it must be treated and
nourished as a unity. It would help if you could hold in the
back of your mind a picture of the *whole* working together
as we discuss the parts.

The general pattern behind all that follows, all that I believe, is *Let's Get Back to Nature's Design and See if We Can
Obey It.* It seems logical to me that the Divine Intelligence
which planned this whole show knew what It was about and
had orderly, sensible methods of maintaining and preserving
same.

Now to particular rules as they have unfolded and worked
out for me:

Get Enough and More Than Enough Protein Daily:

Just how much is that? Well, here's a chart offered by the Food and Nutrition Board of the National Research Council recommending amounts for our daily needs.

AGE		MALE	GRAMS	FEMALE	GRAMS
Adults		"	64	"	55
Teen-Age	20-16	"	100	"	75
Teen-Age	15-13	"	85	"	80
Children	12-10	"	70	"	70
Under 12	9-7	"	60	"	60
" "	6-4	"	50	"	50
" "	3-1	"	40	"	40
Infants.......	1.6 grams per pound of body weight.				

Because they always make these things so easy they add cheerfully that there are twenty-eight grams in an ounce.

Personally, I'm not always a chart man. Sometimes I can't even read them. This one is simply an indication of a scientific minimum. I myself believe in getting more than the amount recommended because this (and most charts) are based on the "normal" adult or teen-ager, etc. under "normal" conditions and assuming that the food in question is A-number-one exactly.

But that's assuming a lot. Many of us aren't "normal" in a nutritional sense because shortages already exist and our "normal" conditions vary under stress and strain (and who today is without these Twentieth Century Twins?) in which case more than normal amounts are required. To assume that a protein is A-number-one, just as evaluated, is difficult because some foods that should contain certain nutritional elements do not, and various methods of cooking can alter what they do contain, as we'll see in Rule Seven. Furthermore, an A-number-one protein is a very specialized thing. Just any old protein won't do.

Here's the snare. When it says so many grams of protein, it means of *complete* or *first-class* protein. And what is this golden nugget? Well, once our protein gets into the body it's broken down in the digestive processes into forms that are absorbed into the blood stream, then reassembled in various combinations to form a lot more kinds of protein especially required by certain parts of the body. These varied protein forms are called *amino acids*.

Authorities currently believe that there are thirty-two amino acids but admit that only twenty-two are out of the mystery class and that only eight of them are essential to our diet. Why? Because *if we get the eight* (some authorities say ten) *essential amino acids our bodies can manufacture all the other*—providing we get them all there daily. If they aren't all there, not only to combine with each other, but with our other food, then a lot of things can't happen and our regeneration scheme is sabotaged from the beginning.

Now, I'm not going to name these eight amino acids, not because I can't, but because it's one set of confusin' details we don't have to be bothered with. It isn't necessary to know the back-flip from the thirty-foot board in order to learn to swim. What is important is to know how to get them in our diet. Here, just for fun, is a list of *complete* or *first class* proteins, those containing not only all the eight essential amino acids, but containing them in balanced proportions to give maximum nourishment to meet bodily needs:

COMPLETE FIRST-CLASS PROTEIN
(Animal—most active biologically)

FOOD	AMOUNT	GRAMS
Brains	2 med. pieces	10
Cheese, American	2x1x1 inches	12
Cheese, cottage	1-2 cup	19
Eggs, whole	2	12
Halibut	1 serving	19
Heart	2 slices	12
Kidney, stewed	1-2 cup	19
Lamb, roast	1 serving	16
Liver, calf, beef, chicken	4 oz.	25
Milk, whole	1 qt.	33
Oysters, raw	4-6	10

Scallops, raw	3-4	15
Shad, raw	1 serving	19
Shad roe	1 serving	12
Skim milk, powdered	1-2 cup	18

The animal proteins, being nearest to human proteins are most "biologically active." Actually, I believe that *at least 50% of our protein intake should come from animal proteins* and if you think this hits your pocketbook, look again at the list. Halibut rates higher than steak and cottage cheese is equal to roast lamb.

And now look back at it once more from another standpoint. It isn't so rough, is it? Nothing "faddy" about cheese, lamb, eggs, or milk, is there? You could even socialize at home, at restaurants, at parties, without appearing odd and still take first class care of yourself.

But obviously, we aren't going to limit our protein intake to the foods listed above, nor did nature intend that we should. It helps in meeting the required minimum to get several servings of *complete protein* daily, but there are also the partially complete proteins and the incomplete proteins, both of which provide good sources that enlarge our dietary horizon and include many of those other necessary materials —vitamins, minerals, natural carbohydrates, and fats.

Here, for example, are some valuable vegetable sources on the list of incomplete proteins:

FOOD	AMOUNT	GRAMS
Almonds	1-2 cup	18
Beans, dried soy	1-2 cup	35
Beans, dried limas	1-2 cup	6
Buckwheat flour	1 cup	15
Corn meal, yellow	1 cup	12
Peanuts	1-2 cup	19
Peanut butter	1-2 cup	19
Peanut flour	1 cup	59
Peas, dried split	1-2 cup	7
Rice, brown	1-2 cup	8.3
Soybean flour	1 cup	45 1
Soybean sprouts	1 cup	8

Sunflower seeds	1-2 cup	35.2
Wheat, whole, flour	1 cup	15
Wheat, shredded	1 biscuit	12
Wheat germ	1-2 cup	16
Yeast, brewer's	1 lb.	45

If I had had that list long ago I might have been a *much* more successful vegetarian.

Partially complete proteins have the eight-count, all the amino acids, but they are not in as perfectly balanced proportions. Incomplete proteins do not have the total amino acid count, but certainly contribute to our over-all protein pattern and should be included in our daily diet.

Here are nature's rules in providing proteins.

> *First, the closer a food protein resembles a human protein the more valuable it will be to us. In everyday menu language that puts lean meats (always including gland meats like liver, heart, kidneys,) as well as fish and poultry high on the list.*

> *Second, all foods meant to produce or nourish new life appropriately enough contain high-grade protein. This includes milk (and milk products), eggs, seeds, whole grains, nuts, legumes (pears, beans).*

> *Third, fresh fruits and vegetables, while listed as incomplete protein sources, nevertheless are a valuable protein addition and should not be overlooked.*

Once again, so you won't weaken before you've given this a try; *proteins come first. Why?* We need proteins in abundance to feed body cells, nerves, bones, tissue, blood, in order to rebuild, replace, repair; to be prepared to defend against any unfriendly intruders. We need protein to form enzymes, nourish glands and supply basic materials for hormones; to regenerate every part of our body until we are truly vital.

attractive, dynamic, healthy, energetic, at any and every age. We need to start getting this material *now, today,* until our body conforms to the pattern nature laid down of Man-As-Man-Should-Be!

How? Get enough and more than enough protein into your diet daily . . . get two generous helpings of complete protein from our list. Try to make half your protein intake animal protein. Include in your diet each day meat, milk, or milk products, eggs, some seed foods, whole grains, legumes, or nuts, fresh fruits and vegetables. Don't worry about putting on weight by following Rule One, especially if you pay close attention to Rules Four and Five.

Chapter 8

Vitamins for Vigor and Vitality

One night when Mary was absent from dinner, number Two daughter, Patricia, assumed her place at the table. Number One son, Robert, who is very grown-up, said, "So you're mother tonight? Well, if you're mother, tell me what are vitamins?" To which pretty Pat replied calmly and without hesitation, "I'm busy; ask your father."

We already have the negative answer of a nutritionist that they "are the substances that make us ill if we don't eat them," and I can add a positive to this. Vitamins are "activators" and they have to have something to "activate," namely proteins, minerals, carbohydrates, fats—which means that you simply can't live on vitamins alone. However, nature put them in food and we get them by eating.

The only two things father could add for Robert were that, stated positively, what the nutritionist said was, if you "get your vitamins daily" your resistance to disease, infection, and physical decay is higher. (Decay is a horrible word, isn't it? But we're facing facts.) And that you'd better "get them all" while you're about it, because if you don't, that *whole* we are keeping in the back of our mind, the body as a unity, is going to suffer in some department. Vitamins promote growth all down the line. They "activate" youthfulness, beauty, the glow of a good disposition, and we will hear more about them as well as minerals and proteins.

Later we'll meet most of them individually and find out their specialty, *where* they come from and *how* to get them into our diet. In connection with vitamins I'd better say right now that I am well aware, as any modern reader must be, of supplements as a means of getting various supplies into our system—and we'll discuss that in detail later. But our primary objective was to "find nature's design and try to follow it." So food comes first because that was nature's original design.

Vitamin A: Among the specialties of vitamin A are normal reproduction of healthy cells, particularly noticeable in the texture of our skin, and resistance to infection. Deficiencies can appear as night blindness and other eye difficulties. Dr. Henry C. Sherman, professor emeritus at Columbia University stated that by eating four times the minimum amount of Vitamin A recommended, man can add another ten years to his prime of life—("prime" I take to mean "feeling good all the way").

Vitamin A is associated closely with the green-pigment plants, the deeper the color, the better. Perhaps the story they tell about Grover Cleveland indicates that he was one of the first advocates of Vitamin A. It seems a lean, ragged man came to the White House lawn and got down on his hands and knees and was chewing grass. President Cleveland from a front window saw the man and asked, "What are you doing?" When the man said, "I'm hungry and have to eat grass," Cleveland reportedly told him, "Why don't you go around to the back yard where the grass is greener?"

There are, however, sources more available to us and just as good even if they don't come from the White House.

> *Besides all deep-green plants Vitamin A is present in liver, egg yolk, cheese, whole milk, butter, all green and yellow vegetables (carrots*

especially!), yellow fruits such as apricots, peaches, persimmons—and also sunflower seeds.

B-Complex: The B-complex is a whole family and, as with the eight essential amino acids in protein, they should *all* be present in our diet. Without them we have lowered resistance and it could almost be called The Personality Vitamin, since a partial deficiency in the B family can result in discouragement, confusion, low morale, depression. It also assists in the formation and maintenance of rich, red blood.

The best general sources for the B-complex family are: leafy-greens, glandular meats, whole grains, brewer's yeast, wheat germ, yogurt; they are also found in meat, fowl, fish, eggs, milk, cheese, seeds, green vegetables, legumes, berries, melons, fresh fruit.

Here are the best known members of the family, and as with all families, we find some have difficult names and even nicknames:

B₁ (thiamin): This is the spark-plug vitamin which must be present before any organism can burn glucose (the form of sugar necessary for oxidation in the body). To get along without it would be comparable to getting along without breathing. B₁ assists in complete oxidation and good assimilation and that, of course, equals vigor and vitality. It is the "pep" vitamin, the absence of which eventually appears as beri-beri, the "I can't" disease.

B₂ (riboflavin): This member of the family is related to skin defects, eye strain, inflamed eyeballs, as well as general health and vitality, since it is needed for enzyme action in breaking down starches and sugars to be transformed into energy. A lack of riboflavin is also associated with skin difficulties.

Niacin: If you don't have this "substance" to a very, very large degree the illness you suffer is pellagra. It is called the "courage vitamin" since its lack seems to manifest even in early deficiency stages as a personality change, a tendency to suspicions, depression, low morale, hostility.

B_6 (*pyridoxine*): This little magician has a soothing sedative effect on the nerves (nature's tranquilizer). It's absence also may manifest as skin disorders, poor muscle tone, dizziness, morning sickness, or nausea connected with various forms of land, air, and sea travel, as well as the growth, texture, and color of hair.

A trio whose names I don't even recommend trying to pronounce, but who still belong to the B-complex family are *Para-Amino-benzoic acid* (nicknamed Paba), *Pantathenic Acid,* and *Inositol*—all of which affect our growth as well as the condition of our skin and hair.

Choline, still in the B-family, along with Inositol, has a bearing on the youthfulness of our arteries and thus on our susceptibility to heart attacks.

Biotin, called quaintly in some circles the "cheerful cherub vitamin" has to do with mental health and with skin tone.

Folic Acid is needed, in small amounts, along with B_{12} and Vitamin C in the production of red blood cells. It appears further to have a connection with the brain itself, hence our alertness and *joie de vivre*.

B_{12} works along with Iron as well as Folic Acid in preventing anemia and a deficiency here is further associated with nerve disintegration.

This does not quite complete the B-complex group. There are a few tag-alongs to this family about which not too much is known and somehow or another new ones seem constantly turning up. But it *is* a powerful as well as a complex outfit, isn't it? It's easy to see why this is a *must* for a happy, healthy body.

Vitamin C (*ascorbic acid*): Like our friend protein, is present in all tissues and cells of the body. It acts as a sort of cement holding the cells together and if our Vitamin C supply is inadequate our minerals can seep away. In children the enamel of their teeth becomes thin. In fact, it is so vital to all our cells and tissues that it is sometimes called the Beauty and Youth vitamin. Along with Vitamin A, Vitamin C is of great assistance in resisting disease and infection. A deficiency here lowers resistance to allergies as well, skin bruises easily and pyorrhea, a soft spongy, bleeding gum condition similar to scurvy, may appear. In an extreme deficiency, of course, we have the bane of the sailor, Columbus' old friend, scurvy itself.

> *Some good sources of Vitamin C: Primarily citrus fruits, raw and canned tomatoes as well as tomato juice, then fresh, uncooked vegetables, melons, apricots, strawberries, persimmons, all green vegetables.*

Vitamin D (the sunshine vitamin): Here is a splendid example of the unity of nutrition to further the unity of the body. Vitamin D is an indispensable member of the Calcium team upon which all our bones, the shape of our faces, jaws, our "skeleton outline" and our teeth depend. We'll meet the Calcium Team again in Rule Three, where we find three minerals, calcium, phosphorus and iodine, working with the Vitamin B-complex, Vitamins D and F (for Fats), and the enzyme phosphatase (enzymes are protein in structure, remember?) to prevent bow legs, rickets, deformed jaws calling for extensive dental correction, all forms of bone deficiencies. Minerals calcium and phosphorus cannot be absorbed into the intestinal tract until sufficient Vitamin D is present. A special duty of Vitamin D seems to be in helping to form the enzyme phosphatase which controls the releasing of phosphorus from fats and sugars so it can combine with the available calcium. We go into this only as an *example* of the interdependence that is going on all the time we are taking these things separately.

The important point to *remember* is that Vitamin D will

help give us strong, youthful, well-shaped bones and teeth, teeth that will last and bones that will knit if broken at any age.

> *The chief source of Vitamin D is sunshine: The ultra-violet rays in the sun activate a substance present naturally in the oil of our skin and slowly change it to this necessary vitamin which is then absorbed directly through the skin. For this reason a daily sun-bath, weather permitting, is a health as well as a beauty treat. The trick is, do not bathe at once if you wish to get the healthful benefits of your sun-bath. Give nature time to work her miracle before you wash off the natural oil.*

> *Food sources are not as satisfactory as sunshine,* since nature didn't design nor foresee how much time you'd spend in a house nor I under a studio arc . . . which is quite devoid of ultra-violet ray. *There is some Vitamin D available in egg yolk, milk, oysters, fatty fish, tuna, salmon, and sardines. But here, if we are not getting enough sunshine, we need the artificial aid of a sun lamp or the concentrated Vitamin D found in fish liver oils (halibut, cod, etc.).*

Vitamin E is referred to by some nutritionists as the number one heart aid, since its presence helps prevent and repair damaged muscles. It assists less dramatic muscles too, according to the late Dr. Tom D. Spies, medical nutritionist at Northwestern University and Hillman Hospital, Birmingham, Alabama. Dr. Spies found that in some cases of muscular inflammation "pain began to ease dramatically in aching backs and limbs" with an increased intake of Vitamin E. This vitamin apparently acts as a blood normalizer as well, since it has proven successful in helping to dissolve blood clots and conversely assists the blood-clotting action for those who bleed too easily. It softens scar tissue, helps heal ulcers, wounds, burns, has—under experimental conditions—improved the muscular power of world athletes and assisted in fertility, successful conclusion of pregnancy and menstrual and menopause disorders. An all-round busy little activator, Vitamin E.

There has developed now the Vitamin-E-complex family with at least six known members and they, in turn, belong to a family group known as the fat-soluble vitamins, all of which work together. Vitamins A, B, D, E, and K, belong to the fat-soluble group; without Vitamin E, for example, Vitamin A (which we have already met as a cell builder) doesn't do its job nearly as well. We mention this here because Vitamin E functions best when in its natural state combined with oils.

> *Thus we find that the Best Source of Vitamin E is in cold-pressed natural vegetable oils, such as olive oil, wheat germ oil, corn and soya oils. It is also to be found, though in less quantity, in sweet potatoes, liver, oat meal, brown rice, turnip greens, and eggs, fish, sardines, and barley.*

Vitamin K is the blood clotting vitamin and *is plentiful in bright-green leaves.*

Vitamin P (*the flavonoids*) have assisted in a dramatic way in helping with all manner of distresses, by "strengthening body defences at a basic level." As simply, or "over simply" as that can be explained—this means that Vitamin P has a favorable action in the capillaries. These capillaries are the "business centers" of our body, for here all the food passes from the blood stream into our cells and tissues and waste products are collected. Vitamin C, as we've seen, is the cement (only it's more like gelatin) that helps hold all the body cells, including the capillaries, together, but there is an additional and very delicate operation here which is de-

lightfully confusing, so please just accept my word for it
that it's vital (or sounds so anyway), and this is performed by
Vitamin P. In this connection, and with the brotherly help
of C, the flavonoids have assisted in stopping bleeding caused
by weakened capillaries, nose-bleeds, or hemorrhages connected with high blood pressure, tuberculosis, etc. With
Vitamin C it has also been of inestimable help in respiratory
infections, from common cold to flu and tonsillitis. Rheuma-
toid arthritis and bursitis have also been helped by this
nutrition magic.

> *Excellent sources of Vitamin P are: Grapes,*
> *lemon, whole oranges, orange juice, orange*
> *peel, prunes, parsley, and spinach. The next*
> *best are apricots, apples, cabbage, cherries,*
> *grapefruit, lettuce, plums, and walnuts. Toma-*
> *toes, potatoes, parsnips, apples, peas, water-*
> *cress, and carrots also contain the flavonoids.*

Vitamin U: This is a sort of unofficial member of the
family named U for ulcers. It was named because Dr. Gar-
nett Cheney of Leland Stanford's School of Medicine gave
thirteen patients one quart of cabbage juice daily. All had
ulcers in various internal organs and all made startlingly
quick recoveries. The vitamin has not, however, been isolated.

> *The best source is, of course, raw cabbage juice.*
> *It is also found in celery, raw milk, fresh, un-*
> *cooked greens, raw egg yolks, cereal grasses.*
> *It never appears in cooked foods.*

There are currently many vitamins still being investigated. One such under my personal experimental observation is known as Vitamin T for Turk. I don't remember
where I heard this, but the story went that, during the campaign in Korea, an extensive medical investigation was made
of the various nationalities engaged with us in this police
action. The objective was to test resistance (or lack of re-

sistance) to "brain-washing." None of our partners, nor we ourselves, faired well. Under expert handling all were susceptible to "brain-washing"—all, that is, except the Turks. Regardless of what was said or done to them the Turks were steadfast, had a superior ability to fix their concentration and stand pat. Results were analyzed and nothing seemed to indicate the reason for this until the matter of diet was investigated. Here it seemed possible that the Turks had access through sesame seeds, which is practically their national dish, to some secret weapon. In Turkey the candy, the flour, the condiment for dipping meat is invariably the same— sesame seed. Thus some of the investigators felt there was a strong possibility that the condition was nutritional.

Now, I wasn't too concerned with my personal ability to withstand brain-washing. But if you have ever raised a young teen-age boy, the fact that anything short of a club could increase his ability to concentrate has untold attractions. Therefore I began my personal experiment on my son, Robert. I am not yet prepared to state whether it is my persuasive personality, the inevitable growth toward maturity, expert teaching in school, or sesame seeds, but Robert is leading his class in all fields after a very slow start.

If he makes the Air Force Academy, currently his largest dream, I shall make my report to the nation. Until then, we'll just have to be satisfied with the proven list above and remember to *get our vitamins daily for vigor and vitality.*

Chapter 9

Minerals Are a Must

With minerals, as with vitamins, we remember that we need only relatively small amounts of each, but we do need *all* of them daily and the difference can tip the scales for us between disease and zestful, exciting health. Also as with vitamins, minerals are closely linked with proteins, with vitamins, and with each other. In many instances they seem to act as *balancers,* helping to keep a body function from going off kilter in either direction. All of them are important in gland functions, all are personality and beauty as well as health aids, and we will hear more about them in their specialties when we come to the "lullaby diet" for tense, high-strung people, and to their intimate connection with the quality and power of your physical attraction and beauty.

Calcium and *Phosphorus* lead off the mineral parade because, we remember, Dr. C. Ward Crampton in his New York report indicated that the American diet was possibly more deficient in calcium than in any other single food element and that it was "one common cause of aging that can be corrected."

We remember, too, that calcium and phosphorus (along with iodine and other trace minerals) plus the Vitamin-B family and vitamins D and F (for fats) and the enzyme phosphatase, are needed to build and maintain healthy bones and teeth. Lime, a form of calcium often found in drinking water that filters through limestone, has provided a natural source of this valuable mineral in states like Texas—where the natives grow noticeably tall and straight and have, as a rule, flashy white teeth.

Abundant calcium together with its assistants will help calm nerves, strengthen and relax our heart and other muscles (muscle cramps, we recall, can be a sign of calcium deficiency), and in turn assist in the calm, quiet sleep that really rests and refreshes.

> *Calcium is found in protein rich foods such as milk, almonds, cheese, and in deep-green leafy vegetables, whole grain cereals, and potatoes.*

Phosphorus plays on another team as well as the one led by calcium. With *potassium* and *magnesium* it comprises a trio which a National Academy of Science research team stated were essential in the diet for all body-building protein foods.

> *Good phosphorus sources include all protein rich foods, meats, cheese, milk, eggs, legumes, vegetables, fruits, whole grains, wheat, rye and oats.*

Potassium, another member of that team also acts as a balancer. A potassium deficiency can lead to constipation as well as slowing growth, but on the other hand has been of great aid in checking diarrhea. Its lack can also manifest as a nervous ailment, displayed as either over-alertness or sleepiness.

> *Foods high in potassium are whole grains, potatoes, leafy greens, vegetables, almonds, fruits, figs.*

Magnesium, the third member of the trio, also relaxes nerves and is needed for normal muscle function. A lack here affects heart, blood vessels, blood pressure. Irritability and nervousness follow.

> *Sources of magnesium: Because it is part of the magic plant substance chlorophyl it is very plentiful in green leaves (the greener the more!). It is also present in nuts, legumes, egg yolk, milk, coconuts, grapefruit and oranges, grain and grain products.*

Iron is boss man of the blood gang, and a vital gang it is. It has had a pretty good press (have you had your iron today?) but not good enough—for current statistics indicate that as much as ninety percent of American women are flirting with anemia in some degree. This, of course, should be of vital concern to the beauty-conscious long before it reaches the stage where the doctor is called, for early symptoms include not only that dragged out feeling, but that dragged out look—limp skin, hair, nails, and poor complexions.

It has a definite effect on sex glands, and that fascinating sparkle that goes with an interest in life and love. Good blood is obviously a prime requisite for female (and male) fascination as well as for healthy life. Not too much attention has been paid to man's predicament on this score, but rich blood is more than a beauty treatment, and the red-blooded American is not always as red-blooded as he should or could be!

Blood is the life-line that carries oxygen, food, blood sugar, and other supplies around the body course. It is made up of plasma (a liquid about the color of straw), white cells (the small warriors that fight off unfriendly invaders), and red cells which transport the magic hemoglobin. (And that is an explanation, I suspect, simplified to the point where the expert will dive two hundred feet and stay there—but it gives the basic idea.) The hemoglobin as well as the red blood cells have an affinity for iron and so, if we have an affinity for health and beauty, we'll provide this mineral together with its working partners. We have already learned that iron needs

the B-complex family for our blood bank, especially Folic
Acid in small amounts and B$_{12}$, plus small amounts of cobalt,
zinc, and other trace minerals which we will meet shortly.
But iron is king!

> *Rich sources of Iron include liver, tongue,
> heart, muscle meats (what a name for steak!)
> molasses, peanuts, apricots, uncooked wheat
> germ, leafy greens (spinach, Swiss chard, pars-
> ley, and mustard greens are particularly good),
> and also fresh fruits, kidney and lima beans.*

Iodine not only works with iron in the blood department
but affects our sexual powers. It is a most important food for
the thyroid gland, the mastermind which is known as the
"pace setter" of the body. We will find later that this entire
operation has much to do with our "silhouette" and the particular spots where we store those unwanted lumps and
bumps. In the personality zone it has a marked effect on our
alertness and manifest intelligence.

> *Best sources of Iodine are sea foods, salt water
> varieties especially, and anything grown in or
> near the sea. Others include garlic, milk and
> milk products, fruits (apples, bananas,
> peaches, cherries) peanuts, carrots, celery,
> seeds and seed cereals.*

Copper is essential to the full use of iron, thus it also helps
prevent anemia and all its train of petty and serious woes.
Again with iron and iodine it is a required material for
healthy sex glands.

> *Copper is plentiful in natural foods, particu-
> larly those containing iron as well—molasses,
> liver, leafy greens, berries, whole grains, plus
> oysters, clams, egg yolk, dried fruit (especially
> apricots and figs.)*

Sodium (*salt to you*): Salt or sodium is mother's little
helper—but a little helps a lot. We remember that salt oc-

curs in the solution of all body fluids and a sudden shortage
from excess perspiration can cause heat exhaustion. It also
gives an assist to the body's use of potassium and calcium, and
is needed to handle carbohydrates. Even if you have plenty
of those eight amino acids (remember?—the complete protein) the synthesis into all the other necessary amino acids
can't take place without salt. Its absence slows growth as
well. But the point with salt is that we get sufficient of it
without half trying—thus it isn't wise unless you are specifically medically advised—to overdo the use of table salt.
Particularly after forty an over dose of sodium is definitely
undesirable.

> *Natural sources of sodium exist in the muscle
> of all animals and in all vegetables, so don't
> reach for more than the usual amount at table.*

Chlorine in California means time to get out and clean
the swimming pool—and in nutrition it follows much the
same idea. Chlorine, that is chlorine as it occurs naturally in
food, because of its cleansing activities in the body and its
use in the digestive juices, has been nicknamed dietetically
"the laundryman." Lack of chlorine can retard growth, cause
fearfulness and apprehension, so it's a mild friendly cleanser
as well.

> *Our best sources of chlorine are table salt,
> raw meat, milk, leafy greens, tomatoes, rad-
> ishes, beets, ripe olives, rye flour.*

Cobalt (as well as *zinc*) works with the Vitamin B complex
plus iron and copper in the formation and maintenance of
blood.

> *The best sources are lobster, buckwheat, mush-
> rooms, carrots, tomatoes, green beans, all whole
> grains.*

Sulphur we mentioned in the last chapter and will mention again later as a beauty mineral. It is a part of that famous
old-fashioned blood cleanser great-grandma recommended

each spring (sulphur-and-molasses—she knew a thing or two, didn't she?) and has a direct effect on skin, nails, and hair.

> Food sources of sulphur include many of the
> protein foods plus cabbage and brussels sprouts
> which have a goodly supply.

Fluorine: Fluorine exists all right—but on the question of its importance and use—the vital question—a fact or fad?—the jury is still out. Therefore, since I decided a long time ago to "accept with gratitude what science establishes as *fact*" I'll wait until the jury is in. For the moment I am leaving it to nature, figuring that, if I get foods high in other minerals, I am doing the best I can. For any questions on fluorine, I bow out. Your dentist is the authority.

Trace minerals include *silicon,* needed for skin beauty, bones, teeth; *zinc,* required by all tissues as well as in the blood bank, plus the thyroid gland and the male hormone (which is also present in the female, I hasten to add, although you'll have to take my word for it, because the explanation is very involved). Zinc is also thought to be needed for the efficient working of Vitamins B_1 and B_{12}; *nickel* and *silver* wanted by tissues and glands; *boron* which helps in cell control; and *bromine,* the so-called "mental health" mineral.

> These trace minerals are present in leafy green
> and all other vegetables, fruits, whole grains,
> meats, eggs, nuts, lentils, legumes.

To sum up Rule Three: These eleven-minerals-plus are a must: *calcium* and *phosphorus* for bones and teeth, *phosphorus, potassium* and *magnesium* "are essential in the diet for all body-building protein foods," *iron, iodine,* and *copper* are the Big Three of the Blood with a necessary assist from *cobalt* and *zinc. Salt* is mother's little helper. *Chlorine* is the "laundryman." *Sulphur* specializes in blood cleansing and beauty while the *trace minerals* are the plus that join the whole mineral family in contribution to beauty, serenity, zest, and a long and happy life.

~~~~~~~~~~~

Chapter 10

Handle with Care

Do you remember Rule Four?

It was *Handle Carbohydrates with Care*.

My personal application of this rule is that *I try to limit my sugars and starches to natural carbohydrates at mealtimes.* The key to this is in three little words: NO EMPTY CAL-ORIES.

Carbohydrates with fats function to provide heat and energy, as we recall, but we don't have to worry about get-ting enough of them because they just come naturally in natural foods.

If you have a sweet tooth (and who doesn't, now and then?) the time to fill it is between meals both for the sake of your digestion and to keep from fooling that appetite into thinking it's been satisfied with building materials when all you've given it was a jolt of "quick energy." Starches or sugars are just not safe substitutes for protein—thus I try to get my mealtime carbohydrates in foods which carry a full load of proteins, minerals, vitamins. Any other mealtime procedure is a little like the wistful performance of the man who had the cabin next to us when we went to Europe.

It was his first voyage and we could hear him, every time the door was opened, groaning with sea-sickness. The second night out we overheard the steward ask if he could send him some dinner. "No," he replied, "just throw it overboard and save me the trouble." If we insist on high sugar and starch meals, empty of the builders, we'd be safer to throw it overboard because it's guaranteed to do us no good and can even do us harm, depriving us of building materials and forcing our body to handle or store more fuel than it can burn.

Remember, we don't have to worry about getting enough sugars and starches. They are present in abundance in natural foods. So for *mealtime energy* stick to the natural carbohydrates found in protein-vitamin-and-mineral-rich fruits, vegetables, whole grains, seeds, and seed cereals. In the full breakdown of meat protein in the body 58% is converted to carbohydrate—so there's another good natural source. Honey, a mineral carrier, is a fine natural sweetener.

To sum up Rule Four—carbohydrates can be friends—or enemies, depending on how you handle them. Handle them with care—natural carbohydrates with meals—treat-time between meals only!

Rule Five: Fats Are Food and We Need a Limited Amount of Certain Fats Every Day. Let's start off by saying that high starch or sugar diets which include fats are dynamite. The damage here from stored fats which are not burned up because we have an overabundance of "energy material fouls our laboratory from top to bottom; thus another reason for handling our carbohydrates with care is to allow room in our diet for the kind of fats which our body urgently needs."

It is unfortunate that the adjective or adverb "fat" used as a personal description is exactly the same as the noun "fat" applied to nutrition—because inevitably people connect the two and the conclusion is obvious. But the real danger of obesity and its ensuing disorders comes from combining an overabundance of empty calories (the *wrong* carbohydrates) with the nutritionally valuable fat foods needed in small amounts as a building material (the *right* fats).

Once again, the basic rule is "Handle with Care."

The proper fats for our purpose are called sometimes by the much nicer name, Vitamin F, since as with vitamins very small amounts of it are effective. Technically Vitamin F comprises the unsaturated, fatty acids without which we can't possibly have the real health, lovely skin and calm nerves we need for fuller living. The unsaturated fatty acids protect those fat-soluble vitamins, A, B, D, K, and E. They contain certain superior growth factors, help adolescent skin problems (as well as yours and mine), and, as we remember, combine with phosphorus to form every cell of the body. Without them we will be "scrawny" instead of "slim." But if taken in the proper quantities, and not in conjunction with an excess of carbohydrates, they will not make us "fat" people.

Again the warning—carbohydrates, when they are over-abundant in our diet, take over that other function of the fat foods, which is to provide first rate energy-fuel, thus allowing the fats to be deposited instead of burned—and we are in trouble. So we must make the effort to handle our carbohydrates with care—and then to get the essential small amounts of Vitamin F we need without fear for our waistline or our health.

> *The best sources of unsaturated fatty acids*
> *(Vitamin F) are natural vegetable oils (cold*
> *pressed, fresh soy, corn, safflower oils etc. which*
> *have not been heated or solidified—and after*
> *making sure they are not rancid! A tablespoon*
> *a day gives us a plentiful supply). Vitamin F*
> *is also found in butter, cream, egg yolk, nuts,*
> *avocados and meats. But these fats are of the*
> *saturated variety.*

To sum up: Rule Five works with Rule Four—Natural carbohydrates only at mealtimes makes room on our menu for natural fats which are a necessary food.

Rule Six: Fluids are fundamental. We must get six to ten glasses of liquid daily, in some form, the exact amount depending on the climate in which we live, our exertion on a given day, and other common sense factors. We agreed that "the foods you eat, the fluids you drink, the air you breathe must supply all the raw materials your cells need etc." In the first five rules we have covered "the foods you eat." The fluids you drink are exactly as important, if not in some respects a matter of priority, for we all know that we could live perhaps two weeks without food, but barely three days without water. Our adult body contains forty-four quarts of liquid and loses about three quarts one way or another on a normal day. The temperature of the body is controlled by water. The blood is 92% fluid. Constipation, dry, withered skin, may be signs of dehydration.

> *Now, we all know that the common source of body fluid is plain drinking water. And water can carry valuable minerals depending on its source. We know too that liquid milk, fruit and vegetable juices are largely fluid as well as being carriers of other fine nutrients. But fresh fruits, leafy and fresh vegetables, potatoes, meats, cheese and bread also contain water.*

To fix Rule Six firmly in our minds let's repeat. Sufficient water, from six to ten glasses daily (or its equivalent) is a fundamental factor in supplying our body's needs.

Rule Seven: Plan, Market and Cook with an open eye on your health, youthfulness and zest for life.

This is the Cummings PMC formula for TLC (Tender, Loving Care) both for yourself and your family. It takes *effort* plus *imagination* to re-make your life through nutrition but remember, without both we'll be right back with Henry fishing in that empty puddle. In the next chapter I've tried to simplify the Six Preceding Rules into bite-size— they'll be sort of capsules I hope will help you find planning easier—and more fun. I have also, to stimulate your imagination and be perfectly honest with you, revealed the few personal "secrets" I've stored away.

One thing you should keep in mind to console yourself if

the initial effort seems up-hill. You didn't develop your present eating habits in five minutes or hours or days. You won't successfully change them all in five minutes or five days either. But you aren't alone while you're doing it. There are a great many people already interested in helping you attain and maintain ideal nutrition.

> *Your doctor is interested in helping you.*
> *Your dentist is interested in helping you.*
> *Your food industries are interested in helping you.*
> *Your Market (super or non-super) is in business to help you.*
> *All nutritionists everywhere, researchers, foundations (a dedicated, dynamic lot!), care more than you can imagine.*

But you have to be willing to be helped.

The medical profession, another dedicated, dynamic and much over-worked group, is interested in *preventing* disease as well as *curing* it and, as we have seen, good nutrition works both ways. If you have specific problems and express a willingness to help yourself through diet, your family physician will be more than willing to cooperate by "stream-lining" your nutritional needs and your supplements to fit your known deficiencies. But many of those I have talked with have grown too discouraged to make more than tentative suggestions along these lines, except in cases of urgent necessity, since their nutritional advice has been so generally ignored. Most of them admit to a lack of belief in many patients' desire to help *themselves.*

E. M. Abrahamson, M.D., referring to physical conditions that respond best to a change in eating habits, confessed honestly that diagnosis and treatment in such cases required pains from the physician and a sacrifice from patients. "Being human," he adds somewhat wistfully, "doctors much prefer to write a prescription for a miracle drug than to order the execution of habits of self-indulgence hitherto considered quite harmless." *

Dentists, by and large, have been among the most courageous pioneers in the science of improved nutrition, conducting experiments, writing books, using their influence to re-convert an apathetic public. Outstanding work in the field of preventive dentistry by proper nutrition has been done by Fred D. Miller, D.D.S., of Altoona, Pa. The results of his nutritional theories are to be seen in the almost perfect teeth of the grandchildren of his first patients. Two of these grandchildren recently made headlines as Pennsylvania's healthiest physical specimens.

The reason for the dentists' crusade is easily understood when we realize that our mouth (condition of teeth and gums) is a prime indicator of the state of our nutritional health. It has been said that if you covered a hundred individuals with blankets, cutting holes where their mouths were, and turned a good dentist-doctor team loose with a flashlight to inspect only that one area, each could give you a pretty accurate description of the health, habits, and probably life span of the subject. In other words, the condition of your teeth and gums is a dead give-away as to the care and respect you have accorded that miracle-laboratory of yours.

The food industries have devoted untold millions of dollars to research and advanced nutritional studies, trying then to offer their best efforts to you, the buyer. *But they must please you to stay in business.* What you choose from the grocery shelves determines what they must supply, hence my advice to you is to *learn to read labels* and buy to feed your body and not your artificially crippled appetite. You'll help them as well as yourself. For instance, a company will offer an improved whole wheat bread or a whole grain cereal de-

---

* *Body, Mind and Sugar,* by E. M. Abrahamson, M.D. and A. W. Pezet. Henry Holt and Co., New York, 1951.

veloped by its nutritionists which is closer to nature's pattern. Side by side with it is the older product of a less informed time. Each item is labeled as to content. The choice of which will be continued, which will be offered tomorrow, is up to you!

If you *market with care,* discuss your meat with the butcher, your vegetables with the green-grocer, inform yourself as to the kind and quality of what he is providing, you are showing an interest in his life's work. We know that vegetables and fruits as well as meat are nature's treasure stores for us: From them we get minerals mined from the soil and obviously the better the soil in which they grew, the richer the minerals mined. Certain locales become famous for certain fruits and vegetables for this one reason. Certain others for meat producing animals that feed on rich pasture. You will find your green-grocer proud of "food-catches"— and your butcher justifiably recommending certain meat, fowl, fish. Make friends with these experts and listen to their advice.

You know already that fruits and vegetables as well as meat must be of good color and texture, must be fresh, in order to give full food value. Vitamins are lost in the "wilting" process and an aged salad or vegetable is just as depleted as an aged tire. So learn to market with as much selectivity and care as you would use if you were buying a new car, or a new dress, or a new sewing machine—*more* in fact, for your car, your dress, your sewing machine, are expendable. They can be replaced. This body is your one-and-only, here and now, so you'll have to make the most of it.

Cooking is primarily a nutritional art—a gastronomical art only secondarily. This doesn't mean that properly cooked foods shouldn't please the eye and palate. They should. But it absolutely defeats nature's purpose in eating to set on the table a dish, no matter how succulent to our taste buds, if it's devoid of nourishment (building materials). Those eight essential amino acids change complexion if over-cooked and some are even destroyed by heat.

Also, everyone knows that high temperature shrinks meat. Thus two identical steaks or roasts cooked by two different methods will come on the table containing different amounts of digestible protein on the care—or carelessness—with which they are cooked.

Meats, to obtain the highest nutrition, should be cooked *slowly, at low* temperature. This conserves proteins, vitamins, minimizes shrinkage, and avoids scorched drippings.

Over-cooking can boil the vitamins and minerals out of the richest vegetable as well. Did you ever pan for gold? You know how all the gold dust settled to the bottom? Well, often in cooking we boil all the "pay dirt" to the bottom, eat the silt, and the nutritional gold goes down the drain, literally.

When it comes to the question "To Cook or Not to Cook?" our household rule is—*half of all fruits and vegetables raw each day.* And we rotate them. In other words, if we have cooked carrots with the pot roast today, and corned beef with cooked cabbage tomorrow, then we have carrot sticks (raw) or cabbage slaw the next time they're served. When our vegetables *are* cooked we use as little water as possible (never any salt or soda in the cooking process) and cook only to an "Oriental crispness," to the point where they still "bite back" as with Chinese peas. Vegetable juices are stored in the refrigerator for use in stocks and stews.

Another good cooking guide is to *learn what not to throw away.* Nutritionally speaking one might say that the biggest pay load in the kitchen of an uninformed cook is the garbage bucket or disposer. Remember those dark green leaves that are full of building materials? Well, what did you do with your tender beet tops last week? Did you know that the outside leaves of lettuce and cabbage have five times the Vitamin B_{12} content of the pale inside leaves? That if you select tender, fresh vegetables you don't need to peel them and you conserve large amounts of the riches nature has stored there for you? That the skin of a potato is a great source of potassium? Unfortunately, while there will be some fuller hints in the next chapter, this cannot be a cook book. There are, however, some fine ones available by nutrition-wise authors. Among these, one of my favorites is "Let's Cook It Right" by Adelle Davis. There are many others, and some of the source books I have listed in the back of this book include menus and recipes. I'll even offer a couple of my own inventions (or is it concoctions?).

But let's cover one more point under the PMC (Plan, Market, Cook, remember?) plan before we move on to these. Frequently I'm asked if good nutrition doesn't "cost a fortune." Let me answer that once and for all. It's up to you. With imagination, careful planning, and that little extra effort on your part it needn't be any more expensive than poor nutrition. Now, I'm not going to deny that currently it's expensive to eat at all. You don't have to be a housewife to face facts—papa still pays the bills. I read a squib the other night from The Controller which said: "To keep us from starving . . . the U.S. Government Printing Office has published just the thing for you—*Recipes for Cooking Muskrat.*" You don't like muskrat? Very well, how about *Directions for Poisoning Thirteen-striped Ground Squirrels?* (Serve with truffles and antidote on the side.)

But there's no need to go to those lengths if you're willing to spend *effort* and *imagination*—qualities of character rather than purse. Make up your mind that every food dollar you spend is going to contribute something definite toward your nutritional health and beauty and vigor. That's being dollar-wise. Then treat your purchases properly in preparing and cooking. That's thrifty, too. No more mangled minerals, devitalized vitamins, exhausted, pooped out proteins. You won't find it expensive and in the long run you'll even save money. Francis Drake, a modern medical doctor, says, "Health is that intangible something that people reluctantly spend a little to retain but which they will spend their last dime to regain once they have lost it."

I should like to knight this medical fellow myself as Elizabeth I did with his sea-faring namesake. For there is a plea to you to overcome your reluctance this minute and spend a little more *of you on you* before it takes your last dime—or before it is too late.

Now we have seven building blocks in a do-it-yourself kit. The next chapter gives us seven ground rules for proper building conditions and then we'll go on to simple instructions on *how* to put all the blocks together. But our Fourteen Rules equal the highest respect and care we can give this miracle mechanism—our body.

Chapter 11

Positive Health

I promised you a fourteen point program that—if you *live* by it—will give you more vigor, vitality and sparkle than you've ever known.

We've had the seven general rules for getting the needed materials.

Now here are the seven rules for maintaining proper conditions.

1. *Sufficient rest and sleep.*

2. *Adequate recreation and exercise.*

3. *Fresh air and sunshine.*

4. *Bodily cleanliness.*

5. *Proper clothing.*

6. *Cooperation with the rules for good digestion and assimilation.*

7. *Due regard for elimination processes.*

Doesn't that look simple? And sensible? Well, it· is. It's nature's design, not mine—and most of nature's designs are both simple and sensible.

It looks simple enough for any grade school student to follow. But it isn't easy for us, the complicated grown-ups, living complicated lives, to adhere to a simple pattern—it's a challenge.

I, personally, found that to get tempo and organization

into my physical habits took a lot of doing. And that ordering life takes, above all, patience, and a belief that it's worthwhile. Let's look at these rules briefly.

Sufficient Rest and Sleep

That means as much sleep as *you* need. Some folks require seven to eight hours, some, like myself, feel fresh and ready to go on five or six hours. Bob Hope maintains a terrific schedule with the help of "cat naps" during pressure days. He'll drop off on a plane for five totally relaxed minutes and awaken with tremendous vitality. If you can afford the luxury of naps—even the five minute variety—take it.

But don't expect your body to give maximum performance on minimum rest, because sleep not only rids us of fatigue but gives the body a chance to restore tissues and go about other important revitalizing business without being called on for any other effort.

Now, if you're always drowsy—even after sufficient "bed rest"—it can be a vitamin deficiency. Check your B complex intake particularly. And give especial attention to the elimination processes. Constipation tends to make us feel sluggish, especially when due to an overabundance of "empty" carbohydrates in the diet.

If, on the other hand, you have difficulty sleeping, tend toward insomnia, well, obviously stimulants will keep you keyed up. And on the nutritional side of combating or preventing insomnia let's note an experiment conducted by Dr. Michael M. Miller, Associate Physician of St. Elizabeth's Hospital, Washington, D.C. He restricted the intake of table salt by insomnia sufferers to 0.5 to 2 grams daily which both helped them to normal sleep and, after a period rid them of disturbing dreams. It's certainly worth a try before the psychiatrist's couch looms.

Calcium we have already observed as a "nerve calmer," and works with *lactic acid* in "sleep chemistry." Cottage cheese, yogurt, and buttermilk are rich in both calcium and lactic acid. Again lack of Vitamin B complex (particularly B, or *thiamin*) can result in troubled sleep as well as drowsiness, for with insufficient thiamin you may be a "sensitive" restless sleeper—awaken at the slightest move, feel there's too much light in the room, sense each twist and turn of the body. Thiamin rich foods include seed cereals (sunflower seeds and millet especially) whole grains, fish, poultry, and gland meats.

Vitamin C also helps you to a good restful night by helping your blood vessels keep their tone, thus keeping circulation flowing to the sleep center of your brain.

Recreation and Exercise

Nature didn't design exercise as something you had to go out and "get" or simulate by various physical distortions. Her design included a great deal of walking, running, manual labor and the like, which stimulated circulation, caused deep breathing, used and toned muscles, melted excess weight, released tensions and such.

Today, to circumvent the labor saving devices which started with the invention of the wheel, we have to put some thought into "getting" our exercise and recreation. But we'll never be at the top of our form until we find a way.

Recreation and exercise can be combined if we give it some thought. And it doesn't really take all that time and money.

Dr. Samuel Clarke used to amuse himself by jumping over tables and chairs.

Dr. Jonathan Swift, English poet, exercised (and no doubt enjoyed it, too) by running up and down the steps of the deanery.

I go walking when I can.

I swim when I can.

When I can't—I "do" exercises.

Exercise and release from tension benefit every part of your body. We are all interested in keeping and bettering our eyesight. Here's an exercise, "The Elephant Swing," worked out for eye re-education technique by Margaret Darst Corbett, which will not only benefit your eyes but relax your entire body.

"Standing with the feet parallel and sufficiently apart for balance, shift your weight from one foot to the other in an easy swaying motion you have seen the elephant use at the circus. As you sway gently from one side to the other, turn head and shoulders with your swing. Let the arms hang limply from loose shoulders, momentum lifting and swinging them free as you turn from side to side. Count aloud rhythmically in tempo with the swing. This is important, because when speaking or singing it is impossible for you to hold your breath. Breath holding is a companion of tension. Deep, rhythmic breathing is necessary for relaxation and for good vision. Rid yourself of the feeling that this swing is an exercise. Think of it as a pleasant surrender to rhythm such as you would give to a waltz. It is relaxing to play a waltz record and hum the tune as you sway.

"Be sure that neck, shoulder, and chest muscles are loose and at ease. Swing all of you to one side, then to the other. Up to the count of sixty you are developing the amount of relaxation you need. From sixty to one hundred, you really indulge in full release of nerves and muscles, every vertebra being loosened, all the inner organs being relaxed. Best of all, the eyes, unbeknown to their owner, begin to shift with their many involuntary little vibrations which bring improved vision. Pay no attention to your eyes; you cannot feel their involuntary motions. You will know when these are taking place, because the entire room will start slipping past you in the opposite direction as if it were a row of railroad cars traveling back and forth. You leave one side, you leave the other side—does the room seem to pass you by?

"Should you feel a bit dizzy, you are 'leaving your eyes behind.' Be sure you get the feeling of *motion* as you swing.

When mind and eyes allow the world to pass by without clinging and fixing on passing objects, car sickness, elevator sickness, and even sea sickness will be a thing of the past. Take all of you, eyes too, from side to side, rhythmically, smoothly, happily as you would do in a waltz. 'Let the world go by.' Do this swing one hundred times in the morning and you will rid your body of any tension that may have been acquired during sleep, for many persons tense while sleeping. Do another hundred swings before retiring and you will sleep so limply that the bed will hold you, you will not need to support the bed." *

But whatever you do—*do something!*

Your body, each muscle and sinew, was meant for use. If you don't want it to atrophy, *use it!*

Fresh Air and Sunshine

This is such an obvious part of nature's plan for us that it really doesn't need any persuasion. Breathing exercises, deep breaths of fresh air, act as a bracing tonic as well as a relaxer. Remember Vitamin D? The best source of—? Right, sunshine on our skin. And today doctors recommend "fresh air" baths for babies because man-as-man-should-be needs to come into contact with the three wonderful elements—air—sunlight—and water. Which brings us to Rule Four.

Bodily Cleanliness

Americans, as a nation, are probably the most scrubbed nation that has existed in the history of the world. We scrub our teeth, our hair, our hides, constantly, so you don't have to encourage adult Americans to bathe. In fact Will Rogers once quipped: "If the father of our country, George Washington, was Tutankhamened tomorrow and, after being

---

* *Help Yourself to Better Sight*, by Margaret D. Corbett. Prentice-Hall; New York, 1954.

aroused from his tomb was told that the American people today spend over two billion dollars yearly on bathing materials, he would say, 'What got 'em so dirty?' "

Me, I'm a shower guy—*but* I do not scrub my entire body with soap daily when I get under that wonderful water, especially if I've been sunbathing.

Most soap removes the natural oils on our skin which, when exposed to the sun, creates that valuable Vitamin D which is absorbed into the body. That magic takes a little time to accomplish and removing the natural oils too soon stops the process.

Natural skin oils also help to keep the skin soft, pliable, and unlined. I remember a beautiful Indian actress with a skin a maharaja would love to touch (or any red-blooded American) who came to Hollywood not too long ago. She was terribly impressed with our extravagant plumbing and horrified that American women "bathe always with soap."

"Did you never try the oil bath?" she asked my Mary.

"Only on the children when they are small," Mary replied firmly.

But truthfully, it made sense. Soap where and when soap is needed. Water, shower or tub, for therapy and refreshment daily (but not disturbing natural oils). And once a week, an all over "oil bath" with a good oil, like we give our infants.

And while we're on the subject of bodily cleanliness, Americans are rightfully conscious of the need for body deodorants and air purifiers in bathrooms. But when the various body odors are too strong it can well be that the inner condition requires attention as well as the outer one.

Usually this indicates that the lower bowel is too alkaline and the correction is to produce a slightly acid condition. Probably the best nutritional method to make this correction is by using a pint of yogurt daily and letting the lactic acid do the work.

Proper Clothing.

In a later chapter we are going to discuss silhouette control
—nutrition wise.

There have been various kinds of silhouette control
through the years from the tight binding imposed on the feet
of the ladies in ancient China which stunted their under-
pinnings until they couldn't walk, to the corsets our grand-
mothers wore which nipped in their wasp waists until they
couldn't breathe.

But it was over seventy-five years ago that one Amelia
Jenks Bloomer became notorious as an advocate of reform in
ladies' dress and appeared publicly in what was then the
scandalous garment which still bears her name. She was the
first of the bloomer girls and started a gradual national strip
tease which wound up for better or for worse in the Bikini.

And, of course, down the years men have shed ringlets and
lace and snuff-boxes until by and large we should all be
dressing *healthfully* if not always *tastefully*.

Yet I know women today who buy their shoes too small
and their heels too high for walking—the very same ladies
who would scorn the lily feet of China. And on my Bob
Cummings' TV show I had all sorts of trouble with silhouette
controllers. Sometimes the girls would come in wearing various appliances which altered their silhouettes in a manner
to defy mother nature's design and make them look deformed. We had to insist on removal of what made them appear top-heavy and/or bottom-heavy (one girl wore a false
bottom until associate producer Eddie Rubin and I insisted
that she get rid of it), as well as those that strapped their
waists so tightly it was impossible for them to talk and
breathe.

A girl would be all out of breath in a scene and I'd say,
"What's the matter?" And she'd say, "Oh, this thing is so

tight!" When I demanded, "What thing?" she'd admit to wearing a "cincher," and I'd say, "Well, go and take it off."

Look, a part of positive health is to have positively the best natural figure possible—but it's positively unhealthy to cinch and squeeze your midriff or pinch your toes. And inevitably it will keep you from feeling vital, vigorous, and at the top of your form.

Dress for eye appeal! But you'll suffer health-wise *and* beauty-wise unless your clothes are sensible as well.

Cooperate with the Rules for Good Digestion and Assimilation

The difference between *diet* and *nutrition* is that diet is the food consumed. Nutrition is the food that the cells of the body utilize.

It is said that Good Diet + Good Nutrition = Health.

It is better said that Good Diet + Good Assimilation = Health.

Indigestion in one form or another is the bugaboo of the modern civilized man. The remedies you get from the drug store are only temporary aids. Yet the permanent solution is simple.

It lies in *understanding how foods are digested:* and *in combining foods properly.* This can be set down in four simple rules.

First, don't overload your stomach. Animals eat when they are hungry. Babies are now given "demand feeding." Three meals a day are fine—but if you snack intelligently between them and at bed time you won't be tempted to *stuff* at the table and give your digestive organs more at one time than they can handle.

Second, eat something fresh (raw) before each meal.

I'm not going to bore you with details but take my word for it, this has a marvelous effect on the digestion.

In the great restaurants of New York's Golden Age, Rector's and Delmonico's, and today in the Stork Club and many nutrition wise neighborhood and hotel dining rooms, a bowl of raw celery and carrot sticks are placed on the table *ahead of the meal*. Fresh fruit cups and raw salads often precede the main meal.

People who know this secret and are aware of the benefits of this digestive magic are sometimes quite put out when it is omitted from a home dinner party menu. In fact, I know a man, an extremist, I'll grant you, but he will actually have a small bite of the center piece if he isn't provided with anything more suitable.

I have actually seen him innocently nibble a gardenia while waiting for his soup.

I honestly don't recommend eating the table decorations and I've never eaten flowers myself (except violets in a salad once at a gourmet affair) but for hostesses who want to protect their table decorations and for those of you who want to assist these digestive processes—try beginning each meal with at least a few bites of some fruit or vegetable in its natural state.

Rule three is: *Do not combine high carbohydrate foods and pure fats at the same meal.* Instead eat your butter or salad dressing (using cold-pressed vegetable oil) with your protein meals. Nature herself combined protein and fats (as in meat and milk) but she never combined it with starches and gave us no method for handling both at the same time.

Rule four—*Eat in Peace—with a smile—on a happy stomach.* And I'm not just being dear old Bob—the Glad Boy. This is sound nutrition—digestion wise!

Deficiencies in body chemistry, as we have seen, influence the mind and emotions. They can make us tired or "lazy," irritable, depressed, sleepless. And your disposition can affect your gastric juices.

Due Regard for Elimination Processes

This is intimately connected with digestion and assimilation—for constipation and diarrhea often are forms of indigestion. Remember the body is an integrated whole, a unity, and if *any* of the five organs of elimination (intestines, kidneys, liver, skin, lungs) are not functioning properly our bodies are not throwing off wastes adequately, a strain is placed on the others, and our vigor, vitality, and appearance will suffer.

We need, for the *kidneys,* an adequate supply of water.

Remember with the *liver*—excessive amounts of nicotine, caffein, DDT, morphine, and atrophin can damage this hard working organ all too easily. Amino acids (protein), Vitamins A & C, and exercise all are aids for liver health.

As for the *lungs,* which expel carbon dioxide and other poisons, they are stimulated naturally by deep breathing (fresh air preferred) and exercise, Vitamins A & C, plus all the other nutrients which build up good red blood, help keep the lungs healthy.

The *sweat glands* in the skin throw off varying quantities of perspiration per day, depending on the weather and the amount of exertion. We must always remember that besides waste, perspiration contains salt, potassium, iron; acids including lactic; and water soluble vitamins B & C; which must be replaced.

Now, the *intestines* give us two common problems—diarrhea and constipation (and it costs America one hundred million dollars a year to try to overcome the latter). One of the chief causes of these difficulties is a too high carbohydrate intake. Then too Vitamin B-complex is urgently needed for healthy function here (and again, yogurt is a good source). Your nerves are prime movers of your bowels and you can look to them to function well from a nutritional standpoint if the supply of B-complex is sufficient. Dehydration is another cause of constipation—so keep your fluids up.

Regularity is an important factor in overcoming constipation. Another secret in preventing this difficulty was recorded years ago when Fraulein von Plessner, a god-daughter of the Kaiserin brought the first kindergarten to America from Germany. She taught her tiny students the secret in simple rhyme:

> When nature knocks at either door,
> Do not attempt to bluff her.
> But hastily obey her call,
> Or you will surely suffer.

To aid in all these functions, elimination, digestion, and assimilation, one big trick is to relax at mealtime. Sit down quietly, compose yourself (Grace at table is sound nutritionally as well as psychologically and spiritually). Don't bolt your food. Take time. Enjoy eating!

Remember it's a ceremony you're performing—an act of reverence to supply the mystery and the miracle of life within each cell of your body.

Chapter 12

Fads, Facts and Food Values

A large aircraft factory near a metropolitan city recently appealed to the Director of Nutrition of the City Health Department. "If you can't give us immediate help," the Personnel Manager said, "we're going to have to discharge a group of workers."

The reason? They were over-weight—over-weight and under-nourished. "They are accident prone," complained the Personnel Manager. "Their rate of illness and absenteeism is high. They are losing their efficiency."

And since weight control is primarily a nutritional problem, in fact the number one public health nutrition problem and the most dangerous—contributing as it does to so many bodily ills, heart trouble, high blood pressure, diabetes, and kidney conditions among them—the Director of Nutrition went into action.

Classes or groups were formed at the factory to educate these people in sound nutrition—which is still the best way for attaining and *maintaining* proper weight. Their jobs were at stake. Their health was at stake. Yet what happened?

After an enthusiastic beginning the attendance dropped off, and those who remained *listened* but didn't *live* the program offered.

Why? Here are the reasons given.

"Too difficult!"

"I get confused."

"I don't have time!"

Now, I've heard those same reasons given in my personal experience. A friend of mine who was not ill but run down beyond just "that old tired feeling," suffering from acute indigestion attacks, headaches, constipation, slight anemia, was given a food value chart by his physician. With it he got a stiff lecture and firm instructions on how to mend his ways.

What was recommended was pretty much what we've covered in our fourteen points. After a week of bored effort, however, my friend told me he found it "too difficult," was "confused," and just had too much to do to bother.

Yet today he has less and less energy with which to do his work. He has become more and more confused by a myriad of fatigue symptoms, and he has even more to do in coping with all his aches and pains.

And the road to positive health just isn't that difficult. Honest!

I've promised that I'd simplify the first six Rules for Flying High into bite size, sort of capsules to help make keeping them easier—and more fun.

You remember the rules—

> ONE: Get Enough and More than Enough Protein Daily.
> TWO: Vitamins Daily for Vigor and Vitality.
> THREE: Daily Minerals Are a Must.
> FOUR: Handle Carbohydrates with Care.
> FIVE: Fats Are Food and We Need a Limited Amount of Certain Fats Every Day.
> SIX: Fluids Are Fundamental.

We then discussed proteins, vitamins, minerals and where to find each separate item. Now, to make things easier, we will reverse this and list the major foods—and the principal values they provide for your nutritional needs.

Foods are as complex in their way as people are. Foods differ in content and quality according to their kind, the soil and climate in which they are grown, and how fresh they may be. In general, however, this list may reveal to you any insufficiencies in your diet, and how to remedy them. Or if there are certain ingredients which you may need in particular, it will show you where to find them.

What we're after is simplification.

We have the Whyness of the Wherefore.

Now we'll try the Howness, by providing a Key Chart to make menu planning fun.

FISH
(salt water
especially)

High Protein
B-complex
Iodine
Sulphur

Special Values
Sardines—Vit. D & E
Tuna   —Vit. D
Salmon —Vit. D

SHELL FISH

High Protein
Iodine
Sulphur

Special Values
Oysters —Vit. C & D
Oysters —Copper
Clams   —Copper
Lobster—Cobalt
Lobster—Zinc

MUSCLE MEATS
(Lean Beef, lamb,
etc.)

High protein
B-complex
Vit. F
Phosphorus

Iron
Sodium
Sulphur
Trace Minerals

GLAND MEATS
(Liver, heart,
kidney, etc.)

High protein
B-complex
Vit. A
Vit. F
Phosphorus
Iron
Trace Minerals

Special Values
Liver—Vit. E
Liver—Copper

MILK
High protein
Calcium
Vit. A

CHEESE
High protein
Vit. A
B-complex

Vit. C
Vit. D
B-complex
Phosphorus
Magnesium
Iodine
Chlorine
Sulphur
Fats
Carbohydrates

Calcium
Phosphorus
Iodine
Sulphur

BUTTER
Vitamin A
Vitamin F

NATURAL VEGETABLE
OILS (COLD PRESSED)
Vitamin E
Vitamin F

EGGS
High protein
Vitamin A
Vitamin D
Vitamin E
Vitamin U (raw)
B-complex
Phosphorus
Magnesium
Copper
Iron
Trace Minerals

POULTRY
(Chicken & turkey)
High protein
B-complex
Calcium
Phosphorus
Iron
Sodium
Potassium

LEGUMES (Beans, peas, etc.)	WHEAT (Buckwheat—Whole wheat)	WHOLE GRAIN CEREALS AND SEEDS
Good protein	Excellent source natural carbohydrate	Excellent source natural carbohydrate
B-complex	Good protein	Good protein
Phosphorus	Phosphorus	B-complex
Magnesium	Trace Minerals	Calcium
Trace Minerals	*Special Values*	Phosphorus
Special Values	Buckwheat—zinc	Potassium
Kidney beans—iron	Buckwheat—cobalt	Magnesium
Lima beans —iron		Copper
		Zinc
		Cobalt

Trace Minerals
Special Values
Oatmeal —Vit. E
Brown rice—Vit. E
Barley —Vit. E
Rye flour —Chlorine

VEGETABLES— LEAFY GREEN	VEGETABLES—GREEN	VEGETABLES—YELLOW
Incomplete protein	Incomplete protein	Incomplete protein
Natural carbohydrate	Natural carbohydrate	Natural carbohydrate
Vit. A	Vit. A	Vit. A
Vit. C	Vit. C	Phosphorus
Vit. E	B-complex	Potassium
B-complex	Phosphorus	Sodium
Calcium	Potassium	Trace Minerals
Phosphorus	Sodium	*Special Values*
Potassium	*Special Values*	Sweet potatoes
Magnesium	Peas —Vit. F	—Vit. E
Iron	Celery —Vit. U	Carrots —Vit. F
Copper	Celery —Iodine	Carrots —zinc
Sodium	Green beans—cobalt	Carrots —cobalt
Chlorine	Brussels sprouts	Carrots —iodine
Trace Minerals	—sulphur	Raw yellow vegetables contain
Special Values		—Vitamin C.
Turnip greens —Vit. E		
Parsley —Vit. P		
Spinach —Vit. P		
Lettuce —Vit. P		
Watercress —Vit. P		

FRUITS	TOMATOES—CITRUS FRUITS—RAW CABBAGE	POTATOES (STEAMED IN JACKET OR BAKED)
Incomplete protein	Excellent source Vit. C	Vitamin A
Good carbohydrate	Incomplete protein	Vitamin C
Vitamin A	Vitamin A	B-complex
Vitamin C	Vitamin P	Calcium
B-complex	B-complex	Potassium
Iron		Phosphorus

Phosphorus
Potassium

Special Values
Grapes —Vit. P
Prunes —Vit. P
Plums —Vit. P
Peaches —Iodine
Bananas —Iodine
Dried apricots
    —Copper
Dried figs—Copper
Cherries —Vit. P
Cherries —Iodine
Apricots —Vit. P
Apricots —Iron
Apples —Vit. P
Apples —Iodine

Chlorine
Zinc
Cobalt
Calcium
Phosphorus
Iron
Sodium
Potassium
Trace Minerals

Special Values
Cabbage juice
        —Vit. U
Cabbage—sulphur

Iron
Incomplete protein

And to help with handling carbohydrates with care, as well as silhouette control later—here is a simple list of the starch content of common fruits and vegetables:

0% Vegetable—Mushrooms

3% VEGETABLES (LOW CARBOHYDRATE)

Asparagus	Cucumbers	Endive
Kale	Leeks	Celery
Rhubarb	Spinach	Egg plant
Cauliflower	Swiss chard	Lettuce
Tomatoes	Cabbage	Watercress
Olives	Greens	

6% VEGETABLES & FRUITS (LOW CARBOHYDRATE)

Vegetables	*Fruits*
Kohlrabi	Cantaloupe
Okra	Watermelon
Peppers—green	Avocado
String beans	Strawberries
Broccoli	

9% VEGETABLES & FRUITS (LOW CARBOHYDRATE)

Vegetables	*Fruits*
Beets	Cranberries
Carrots	Gooseberries
Onions	Grapefruit

Oyster plant (salsify)
Parsnips
Peas (canned)
Rutabagas
Squash—Hubbard
Squash—Acorn
Squash—Baking
Turnips
Brussels sprouts
Pumpkin

Limes
Muskmelons
Oranges
Lemons
Honeydew melon

15% VEGETABLES & FRUITS

Vegetables

Peas, fresh (green)

Fruits

Apples
Apricots
Blueberries
Blackberries
Cherries
Currants
Grapes
Huckleberries
Loganberries
Mulberries
Nectarines
Orange juice
Pears
Pineapple
Plums
Peaches
Raspberries

20% VEGETABLES & FRUITS

Vegetables

Beans (dried or canned)
  lima
  kidney
  navy
Brown rice (cooked)
Corn
Potatoes—white

Fruits

Bananas
Grape juice
Figs (fresh)
Persimmons

30% VEGETABLES & FRUITS

Vegetables

Potatoes (sweet and
  yams)

Fruits

Apples (dried)
Prunes (fresh)

70% FRUITS

Dried fruits

Apricots
Currants
Figs
Peaches
Pears
Prunes
Raisins

Putting the Blocks Together

Now, knowing what we know about the human body's needs—we can look at the Key Chart of Basic Foods above and see how to plan and prepare meals that meet them.

Nutritionists originally attempted to convince the public by means of a daily "Basic Seven" Group of Foods. The U.S. Department of Agriculture Nutritionists recommended that you include in your meals each day the minimum number of servings from each of the following groups. Teen-agers and very active adults should have extra-large servings.

1) Leafy, green, and yellow vegetables (raw, cooked, frozen, or canned): 1 or more servings.

2) Citrus fruit, tomatoes, raw cabbage, salad greens, raw cantaloupes, pineapples, and strawberries: 1 or more servings.

3) Potatoes and other vegetables and fruits: 2 or more servings.

4) Milk, cheese, and ice cream: 2 or more cups milk (adults): 3 to 4 cups milk (children). Cheese and ice cream may be substituted for one cup of milk.

5) Meat, poultry, fish, eggs, dried beans and peas, and nuts: 1 serving of meat, poultry, or fish, if possible; 4 or more eggs a week; 2 or more servings of beans, peas, nuts and peanut butter per week.

6) Bread, flour, and cereals: some each day.

7) Butter and fortified margarine: some daily.

You can see how, if these were taken in adequate amounts daily, properly prepared, properly combined, such a diet should start one on the road to vim and vigor.

Recently the Agricultural Research Service of the United States simplified this even further in a pamphlet called, "Essentials of an Adequate Diet." The Service proposed the Essential Four daily food plan. It tallies very well with the earlier suggestion we quoted from Dr. Charles E. Dutchess as to the necessity of eating "plenty of lean meat, eggs, milk, vitamins and minerals obtained from a broad selection of meats, fruits and vegetables." Here are the Essential Four.

1. Bread-cereals group:

Four or more servings. Bread or cereals—enriched, whole grain, restored.

2. Meat group:

Two or more servings. Beef, veal, pork, lamb, poultry, fish, eggs with dry beans, peas and nuts as alternates.

3. Vegetable-fruit group:

Four or more servings including: A dark green or deep yellow vegetable, important for vitamin A—at least every other day; a citrus fruit or vegetable important for vitamin C—daily; other fruits and vegetables including potatoes.

4. Milk group:

(Including cheese, cream, butter, etc.)

Commenting on this plan, Fred V. Hein, Consultant in Health and Fitness, American Medical Association, wisely wrote:* "Of course it is next to impossible to devise a nutrition blueprint that is just right for everyone. Needs will obviously differ in terms of age, sex, amount of physical activity, and differences in the use of food within the body. But the 'Essential Four' offers a *minimum food plan* which can be adjusted individually to meet specific needs."

---

* *Journal of Health-Physical Education-Recreation*—March 1958 (Copyright 1958 by The American Association for Health-Physical Education-Recreation, National Education Ass'n, 1201 166 St., N.W., Washington 6, D.C.).

The italics are mine.

As early as 1941, our Federal Government established and published in the Federal Registry that certain Vitamins and Minerals are essential to human nutrition. A Minimum Daily Requirement was established for some. Since 1941, some have been added as scientific research directed.

Minimum means the *least* we can get along with to just get by.

Daily means that we must have them *every day*.

Requirement means that we *need* them.

Now, I just don't believe that, if we really want to reach and maintain the top of our form physically we can take a chance on a *Minimum Food Plan,* or a Minimum Daily Vitamin and Mineral Requirement. With many of us some deficiencies already exist. We have some catching up to do. Then, too, during certain seasons of the year some fresh vegetables and fruits are in short supply leaving a possibility for insufficiency even with the aid of the frozen and canned varieties. Careless cooking outside the home can dissipate necessary vitamins and minerals. Sometimes older people, "sot in their ways," can't be persuaded to the Essential Four let alone the Basic Seven. And the young aren't young enough to be either force fed or old enough to be entirely trusted to get them away from home.

The average person finds himself traveling more and more —by train, boat, plane, helicopter, and in many places where he has almost no control over quality, quantity, or honesty of the food he consumes. Besides, all of us—not just grandpa and junior—are creatures of habit who eat by *choice*—and quite often the whimsical freedom exercised in "choosing our favorite repast" leaves all kinds of chinks in our nutritional armor.

Even with intelligence and common sense, those of us traveling and on the move can't have these wonderful seven basic foods fresh on our own table.

In all such cases certainly a well balanced complete Vitamin and Mineral Food Supplement is in order and you will find many doctors today recommending them *just to be sure*.

But since our primary plan in this book was to "find nature's design and try to follow it," I will now let you in on those few secrets I've tested over the years that deal with nature's own treasure houses.

They're not Top Secrets in the world of nutrition, I'll admit. A lot of dedicated people spend a lot of time trying to spread the word.

They're not fad foods, either.

They're just good sound tips from me to you on how to raise your basic food plan from *minimum* to *maximum* so that you can be fully alert and vibrant with physical well being.

Fads, Facts, and Food Values

The "food faddists" have been taking quite a ribbing lately.

Larry Gelbart, a TV writer, recently reported to a Paris pal that Hollywood was on a "new kick."

"Instead of food," he said, "they're eating dandelion hearts, roots of moss and Eucalyptus bark. It's very dangerous to be invited to someone's house for a meal. For one thing, you can't walk on their lawn because that may be your dinner."

And, he claimed, when the butler announces "dinner" you're apt to get "boiled peanut water, wheat-germ pancakes, soy beans cooked in their own soy, carrot salad and cider vinegar."

The columnist, Cassandra, goes Larry one better in expressing mock jubilance over a manufacturer's announcement of "a complete food—a single food that can support human life." He describes the imaginary dialogue of a normal host with a "complete food" faddist guest.

"Can I tempt you to our asparagus omelette?" asks the host.

"No, thank you. Just a dash of pantothenic acid," says the faddist.

"Or, perhaps, my specialty, carp in mushrooms, herbs, and cooked in wine, oil, butter, with a haunting parsley sauce?"

"What I really go for is a good plateful of choline in delicious powder form."

"Would you care to try our young carrots cooked in Burgundy?"

"Got any phosphorus with just a dash of iodine? I love that gritty flavor."

Now, I invite Mr. Gelbart to walk on our lawn any time, and promise him we *never* cook our beans in their own soy. And as for the "complete food," well, in all my experimenting I've never found a practical one, although I'll admit I've tried.

The search for one complete food is nothing new.

Vasari, in his lives of the painters, describes how Piero di Cosimo, finding that eating interfered with his work, took to living entirely on hard-boiled eggs. He cooked them a hundred at a time, and kept a basketful beside his easel. "That," comments Aubrey Menen, "is one way of simplifying the pursuit of beauty." But it is not, I hasten to add, the way to simplify the problem of how to stay young and vital.

As recently as a few months ago a young friend of mine, an ambitious and dedicated woman writer, read somewhere that papaya was a "complete food." She dashed to our famous and fabulous Farmers' Market and bought a crate of papaya, intending to live solely on this magnificent and valuable fruit, save herself the distraction and bother of PMC (planning, marketing and cooking) while she dedicated herself to her art.

Fortunately, she discovered she just didn't *like* papaya.

Fortunately, because, here again, she would have found that far from simplifying her problem, her vigor and vitality would *not* have been completely nourished on papaya alone.

So far as I know there is no miracle, cure-all complete food;

no magic sprout or bark or pill that can replace a sensible, balanced diet.

The closest anyone has come to a nutritionally successful, uniform, simple diet is Vilhjalmur Stefansson, the explorer-anthropologist, and his colleague, Karsten Andersen. In 1912 under the observation of a host of medical experts at the Dietetic Ward of Bellevue Hospital, including Dr. Eugene F. Du Bois, later Professor of Physiology at Cornell University Medical College and Chief Physician of New York Hospital, these two men undertook to live for a year on nothing but meat.

This was a diet on which they had seen the Eskimos, a Stone-Age people, live and thrive. In the Arctic for ten winters and many summers, Stefansson himself had lived among the Eskimos on a diet of meat (both the lean and fat) and water.

At the end of the experiment both men were in excellent health, slightly better than when they started.

Twenty-seven years later, in 1955, Stefansson, unable to shed ten pounds as ordered by his doctor decided to return to the "stone age meat and fat diet."

"They (the Eskimos) were the healthiest, happiest people I have ever known," he told his wife, "and during ten years among them I never saw a fat man, woman, or child."

His wife, Evelyn, reporting on the results (in the introduction to "Eat Fat and Grow Slim")* wrote:

"How does one measure the miracle of a return to exuberant health? That was the happy result for Stef some months after embarking once again in 1955 on his all-meat diet."

This diet, she reports, enabled him to lose approximately one pound each week until, in seventeen weeks, he lost seventeen pounds. He began to lose weight almost as soon as he started this diet, but after losing seventeen pounds he lost no

---

* *Eat Fat and Grow Slim,* by Richard MacKarness. Doubleday & Company, Inc., New York, 1959.

more and his weight thereafter remained relatively constant. But there were other, and more interesting results.

At this time, Stefansson had passed his 75th year and he was bothered by stiffness in a knee and soreness in hip and shoulder. To favor his knee he made it a practice on stairs to take them one step at a time.

"One day," his wife reported, "some months after the start of our meat diet, he found to his surprise that he could use both legs with equal facility in climbing the stairs. Astonished, he proceeded down. When he had reached the foot of the stairs, without pain or stiffness, he shouted for me to come and see."

Nutritionally, this seemed to be a "complete food" for Stefansson, proving my dad's point that man is protein.

But for the average person (of which I am one) this *could* become monotonous *and* expensive, even if the cheaper cuts of meat, particularly mutton (which the Stefanssons learned to enjoy at 19 cents per pound, the whole mutton) are used.

My tips will combine variety, natural nutritional supplements, and inexpensive protein for those who want to stay vital the easy way and avoid extremes or fads.

First—I eat seeds and nuts between meals. Sesame seeds. Millet. Sunflower seeds. Almonds. Peanuts. Raw. Unroasted. Just like Poor Polly, the parrot. Or the circus elephant. I carry them on the set at the studio. I have a pack or two in my pockets on personal appearance tours and when traveling, for that extra lift. And I like them.

Peanuts, almonds, millet, sunflower and sesame seeds are, you remember, a good source of protein. Seeds and nuts also contain valuable vitamins and minerals.

Peanuts, almonds, sesame and sunflower seeds are palatable as well as nutritious. The taste of millet—I won't fib to you— is dry and boring. But it can be added to your breakfast cereal. Or you can do as I do and just "take it."

Here are lists of the main goodies packaged for you by nature in seeds and nuts:

SEEDS

Sesame	Sunflower	Millet
High protein	*High protein*	*High protein*
B-complex	B-complex	Vitamin A
Calcium	Vitamin D	Vitamin E
Phosphorus	Iodine	Phosphorus
Iron	Lecithin	Iron
Trace Minerals	Magnesium	Magnesium
Vitamin T	Phosphorus	Trace Minerals
(for Turk or	*Iron*	Potassium
Think: and being	*Calcium*	Copper
investigated by	Silicon	Sodium
B. Cummings)	Fluorine	Vitamin F
Vitamin F (unsat-	Vitamin F	
urated fatty acid)		

NUTS

High protein
Calcium
Phosphorus
Iron
Sodium
Potassium
Magnesium
Trace Minerals
Vitamin F

Unblanched almonds	Roasted peanuts
Good protein	Good protein
B-complex	B-complex

My second tip is: *Add powdered skim milk, wheat germ, and Brewer's yeast* to suitable dishes and drinks when preparing meals.

All three of these items contain *good protein* (all the amino acids). Three-fourths-cup of powdered skim milk has all the nutrients that are in a whole quart of fresh skim milk. It can be tolerated by many who can't drink fresh milk.

Brewer's yeast, the de-bittered kind you can buy today, and wheat germ, are a great natural supplement in cooking— added to stews, cereals, soups, etc., they boost not only the protein content, but the vitamin and mineral value as well.

Here's what you get in the Big Three:

WHEAT GERM	BREWER'S YEAST	POWDERED SKIM MILK
Good Protein	Good Protein	Good Protein
B-complex	B-complex	Calcium
Iron (raw)	Calcium	Phosphorus
Calcium	Phosphorus	Iron
Phosphorus	Potassium	Sodium
Sodium	Nicotinic acid	Potassium
Potassium	Iron	Vitamin A
Vitamin C	Sodium	Vitamin C
Vitamin A		B-complex
Nicotinic acid		

My third tip is: *I try to eat liver in some form at least three times a week.* And I don't believe in cooking it to death (the death of its vital protein, vitamins and mineral content).

Calves liver is preferred by most people from a purely gourmet standpoint—but pocketbook wise, baby beef and chicken liver, if carefully prepared, can suit the most discriminating palate.

When an animal has excess nutrition it is stored up chiefly in the liver, so when you or I eat this gland meat it is as if a rich man died and left a lot of money in the bank to us.

Liver is not only a source of *complete protein,* but contains *important* amounts of most vitamins and minerals:

LIVER

Complete protein
Vitamin A
B-complex
Vitamin C
Calcium
Phosphorus
Iron
Iodine

The story is told that when a friend saw the eminent vegetarian, George Bernard Shaw, taking liver, the friend said, "Why, Bernard, I thought you were a vegetarian."

"I am," said Shaw, "this is my medicine."

My fourth tip is: *Be sure to eat some of your fruits whole. When you do—eat skins and all where possible. With such fruits as oranges, pare, don't peel them.*

Fruit juices are good for you. But in my opinion they can be overdone. The reason—first, because fruit juices are *so* good, and *so* easy to drink, that you can down a good deal more on a hot day than you need and I think that throws your sugar balance off. That's my personal opinion and there are probably as many nutritionists who *disagree* with me as there are who *agree*.

But the second reason is that whole fruit is good for you. There are some very fine nutrients and valuable roughage in the parts the "juicers" throw away.

Therefore, I say, be sure that fifty per cent of your fresh fruits are whole, skin and all when palatable, and when you want to remove the skin, *pare, don't peel*. With an orange, leave some of the white that lies between the fruit and the skin. It's good for you!

Imagination and Nutrition

I don't want anybody to get the idea that eating ceases to be a gastronomic joy if you "do it right."

I don't want to give you the idea, either, that I personally just think of my proteins and grimly munch millet seeds.

Quite the contrary.

Around our house we consider it a great challenge to the creative sense to create exciting meals that keep us all, from tiny Tony to father Bob, in top shape.

We use the material provided in this chapter, the Key Chart, *plus* nature's supplements, *plus* imagination and you'd be surprised what we come up with.

For instance, just thinking about it while I'm writing, I've *created* a Cummings Cocktail—powdered skim milk, water, a raw egg yolk, a dash of Brewer's yeast, a ripe banana (for flavor as well as nutrition) and maybe a little honey—(natural honey has *minerals* as well as sweetness to recommend it). Time out while I try it!

— — — — — —

It's tasty.

It's nutritious. (Check the Key Chart and the nutritional values of powdered skim milk and Brewer's yeast and see for yourself.)

I've got a feeling I can alter its flavor by varying the fruit. But it's fun. And Mary, who isn't here right now, will probably have something to add.

Or how about a Scintillating Salad? With *raw* vegetables (dark leafy green—lettuce, very young spinach, watercress, etc.) plus strips of cheese and meat left over from the roast, *plus* a dressing of cold pressed vegetable oil? Or fruit (raw, whole, and a few raisins and dried apricots), on a nest of dark green leaves and topped with yogurt or sour cream dressing?

Check those on the Key Chart.

Soups and stews, scrambled eggs, omelettes, almost anything you care to name can be brought to a new high nutritionally if you *use your Key Chart plus imagination plus the riches nature has stored up for you.*

This, then, coupled with *living* our fourteen points, is the simple secret of what constitutes the highest respect and care we can give that magnificent super-laboratory, the human body, and the nutritional basis for staying attractive and vital for the full span of a long and happy life.

꧁꧂

Chapter 13

Are You Lop-Sided?

You will remember that it was my physician father who first convinced me of the necessity for "knowing myself" *nutritionally* if I wished to live a healthy, happy, successful life.

And that my experiences have led me to believe that he was *one-third* right.

It was my minister mother, many years later, who convinced me of the necessity for "knowing myself" *mentally* and *spiritually* if I truly wanted an all-round healthy, happy, successful life.

The day my mother decided to become a minister in the Church of Religious Science, I thought it was a great thing—for her! From the time of my father's death until that moment, she had seemed to live only half a life. Religion, I thought, was just what she needed.

I had no idea that I needed it as well, nor that, through her study, I would discover that I was lop-sided.

Already I'd done a heap of living up to that point, gay, adventurous living, a sort of balancing act on the tight rope woven, as I mentioned before, of mad deceptions that might break at any moment and tumble me into oblivion, if nothing worse. In the years between the day I donned my first make-up on Broadway and the day of my mother's decision, I had perpetrated not one, not two, but *three* successful masquerades on the sharpest experts as well as the unsuspecting public. These had nothing to do with the roles I played on stage and screen. They were *me,* the guy I went home with every night.

For the first five years of my theatrical career I, Charles Clarence Rôbert Orville Cummings, of Joplin, Missouri, was an Englishman named Blade Stanhope Conway. Then literally overnight I transformed myself into Bob Cummings of San Angelo, Texas, and just as I was getting around to Joplin and home, I became the heir to a mythical fortune from a very real mountain my gullible dad had bought in Nevada. I remember those headlines yet: "Joplin, Mo., Kid Becomes Millionaire."

How did all this happen?

It was simple. I told the first lie. The others followed almost automatically. And that first lie, as usual, could be explained so logically.

I gave up college and dreams of being an aeronautical engineer when the depression, plus my dad suffering a heart attack, practically put me in the bread lines. Why I elected to stand in the actor's bread line in New York is not quite clear to me even yet but it had to do with the friendly persuasion of my college roommate. In 1931, Broadway was surviving by importing risk-free British plays complete as they had succeeded in London. There was a great demand for British actors. I was starving. At the point where I'd eat any old free carbohydrate and hunger can be the mother of invention. Ergo! I would become a British actor.

This necessitated cashing my one asset, a small insurance policy, making a cut-rate round trip to England in the bowels of a tossing ship, and spending my allotted twenty-nine days in the British Isles using a thirty-five dollar motor-cycle for transportation, feverishly acquiring a British accent, British clothes, from underwear to umbrella, and mailing my own advance publicity from Southampton to New York the day I sailed for home.

On my arrival, Mr. Blade Stanhope Conway, that young

"English author-actor-manager-director-producer not interested in money but desiring experience in the American theater" was snatched immediately past the bread lines and I was given my first part in the theater.

Oh, I was a gay deceiver! And I could rationalize so easily. Didn't many theaters advertise "Fifty beautiful girls" when there were no more than twenty-five and only half of those "beautiful"? Weren't sword swallowers and Latin lovers billed as the Sheik of Samarkand when they had probably never traveled past Poughkeepsie? When the butterflies fluttered in my stomach, and they did flutter, I would try to remember the sword swallowers and forget my father's face. My dad, besides being a very fine doctor, had been *radical* with me about telling the truth. While he was not religious in the accepted sense, he had always assured me that *"the innermost becomes the outermost. If you have a tricky personality, it will show in your face."*

But if I thought my face was looking odd, or I felt sad about the passing of Charles Clarence Robert Orville Cummings, his repudiation of his kith and kin and the townfolk of Joplin, and his adoption by a host of English relations, or his precarious position as an English "author-actor," I would look at Blade Stanhope Conway's bank book and feel comforted.

From a Galsworthy play right through to the Ziegfeld Follies I went on weaving my skeins of deceit, trying to remember my lines off stage as well as on, until one fine day four years later, I found myself caught in my own web.

I couldn't get a job because I was "British." I tried New York. I tried Hollywood. The depression was over and with it the need for imports. My Hollywood agent finally told me the bitter truth. "We've got to drop you, old boy. English actors are a drug on the market."

I wailed. I really wailed—and spent a whole afternoon trying to resurrect the American me. My father was gone now, and mother was living in Hollywood almost as a recluse.

Nevertheless, I took my agent to call on her. I dug out my American passport which had been carefully concealed all these years. I tried valiantly to recover my Missouri twang. "I'm not English," I kept saying frantically in a decidedly British accent, "I just talk like an Englishman."

"Amazing," said my agent, finally convinced that I was indeed none other than C.C.R.O. Cummings of Joplin, Missouri. And I knew one whole hour of sweet release. But only one hour. Then my agent called in high excitement. "Forget that Joplin bit, kid," he said, "by tomorrow morning you're from Texas."

It was, he informed me, a very good part, but it had to be the real thing, a genuine lad from Texas. And the director, King Vidor, who was insisting on the McCoy, was a Texan himself. I had had twenty-nine days to transform myself into an Englishman. In fourteen hours, working all night long, I shed my ancient British lineage and broad A, and acquired a hard-working family, a ranch in San Angelo, Texas, plus a toothpick and a slow drawl.

It worked. And so began my second masquerade. This time I was a not-so-gay deceiver. There were no bread lines and I hadn't planned this. It just sort of happened. Besides, I developed a great admiration for King Vidor and lived in constant fear that he would find me out or that someone who had known Mr. Conway would see through that slim toothpick.

My guilty conscience showed every time King Vidor said, "The greatest assets an actor can have are kindness and honesty; *particularly honesty. You can't trick the camera. It sees into your very soul.*" Or I would feel he was looking straight at me when he repeated his favorite quotation from Thackeray: *"The world is a looking glass and gives back to every man the reflection of his own face."*

I'd console myself with the thought that I wasn't hurting anyone but myself. The trouble was I didn't know just how true that was, nor how much I was beginning to hurt.

Then came an agonizing hour when we were almost through with the picture and someone saw through the toothpick. Not a word was said but when I sat beside King Vidor to view the daily rushes of the kid from Texas, suddenly on the screen flashed a test made of Blade Stanhope Conway, from the Lives of a Bengal Lancer.

"Amazing," said Mr. Vidor. "How do you do it, and which one is you?"

"Neither," I said shamefacedly. But I stayed a Texan because the publicity was out. And pretty soon, there I was again, caught in my own web. My range was limited. I could only play southern parts. The burden was getting heavier.

Meanwhile, mother had started going to church and attending lectures. And I would take her. My private life at that point wasn't very satisfactory. It was a sort of reflection of my own confusion. A shadow, a fantasy, can't have a very *real* life. There wasn't any *real* me for it to happen to. This much I began to understand. Finally one day I walked into the studio publicity office and announced: "I want to be *me* even if it wrecks my career." Then I told them my story.

I walked out feeling much better. I thought I was free. But I wasn't. Not too long after that I heard that I was going to be dropped by that studio. It gave me quite a jolt and I retreated into my old pattern. Immediately I thought of some worthless paper in an old trunk mother had had sent out from Joplin, title to half a mountain my father had bought in Goldfield, Nevada. "There's gold there, too," mother had said. "And once I was approached by some lawyer about buying it. But the others couldn't agree on a price and besides, I don't think they've found a way to get the gold out profitably."

Well, that didn't even phase me. I thought it would be more fun to quit as a millionaire than to be dropped as an actor. So I purposely let hints fall in all the right places. The results—headlines: *"Joplin, Mo. Kid Becomes Millionaire."*

Suddenly, I was horrified. It seemed as if the deceptions

were now operating the deceiver. *How* had it happened? *Why* had I done it?

It was then that my mother began studying for the ministry. The more she learned, the more she talked about it, and the more I learned. I began to see "why," and how much I was hurting myself. By constant denial of myself the inner had indeed become the outer. My outer world was reflecting my own guilts and fears, I didn't believe in myself any more or in my talent unless I pretended it belonged to someone different because I had constantly rejected the *me* that God created.

It didn't seem to make any difference whether you started with a Little White Lie about having gone to college when you barely got through high school, to bolster your self esteem (which wasn't a problem with me since I managed several years of college before my father's illness made further schooling impossible) or a Gay Deception like Blade Stanhope Conway, to bolster your bank account. You were actually starting an unholy stream of errors that multiplied until they weighed you down *mentally, spiritually* and *physically.*

For I was suffering physically. My health, weight-wise, cold-in-the-head-wise, fatigue-wise, was going up and down on a see-saw just like my career, no matter what I ate. Now I was high. Now I was low. Nothing would stabilize.

And then, one night, my mother and I had a long talk—about "the unity of man"—the trinity that is unity. We agreed that man is *one,* body, mind, spirit. And that each affects *all.*

I already knew the truth of the body's influence on the mind and spirit and life as a whole, that as Karl B. Mickey said, "where physical stamina is lacking the will lacks power; and the process of thinking . . . is profoundly influenced by the state of general health."

In order to make converts to the cause of nutrition among my religious friends I had often quoted St. Francis de Sales:

"The spirit cannot endure the body when over fed but, if underfed, the body cannot endure the spirit."

Now I had to recognize that to integrate my life I had to accept just as wholeheartedly the effect of the mind and spirit on the body and life as a whole.

Man is a tri—unity.

Each facet affects the whole.

I had been concentrating on one facet—nutrition. Unfortunately, just as the laws of poor nutrition will affect the ignorant along with the informed, so the laws of poor thinking had gone right on affecting me, whether I was aware of it or not. I was lop-sided.

I had been too busy pretending even to begin any voyage of self discovery in this department. I had been mentally denying me as God made me—and accepting a confused pattern based on myths. Once I saw a dynamic change in *thinking* and *doing* as part of the Great Adventure, I was willing to start at once.

The studio did drop me, despite my phony millions, before I could quit. And when I went to a new studio I walked right into the publicity department and said: "This time I tell it straight. I'm now Bob Cummings, no accent, no millions, and I stand or fall on that. I've spent too many years of my life walking a tight rope of twisted stories. Here's where I cut the rope."

The greatest things in my life, my marriage to Mary, our family, my TV career, plus the peace of mind so essential to positive health, all these have come to me since I learned that, while you are what you eat—you are also what you think and what you pray.

And I would be telling you only one-third of the truth of how I believe we can stay young and vital and successful if I didn't share these beliefs with you. However, let me say this —if I had it to do all over again I'd use a system of positive thinking that I now know to be a true religion.

You can have anything you want by acting—acting with all your heart as if you already have it.

This means if you put yourself in the physical and mental positions of happiness, vibrant health, wealth, and good fortune, and really believe with all your heart that you already have attained them—you will. The secret is blind belief.

Christ said, "What things soever ye desire, when ye pray, believe that ye receive them, and ye shall have them."

Chapter 14

Positive Living

The sciences of medicine plus nutrition and biochemistry have proven conclusively that *what you eat, or don't eat,* affects not only the body but the mind and spirit. Irritability, anxiety, depression, lack of will power and brain power, laziness, and a myriad other so-called "defects of character" can stem from improperly nourished, poorly cared for, bodies.

Now, to get the *whole* picture, we have to reverse this.

The sciences of medicine, particularly psychiatry, plus psychology, have proven that *what you think and feel* affects the body. Psychosomatic symptoms are physical disturbances that can be traced to emotional causes.

Negative emotions, hate (including resentments, quarrels, and all such variations), fear, guilt, inferiority feelings, can churn up our internal workings, forcing tensions, over-working glands, and generally creating chaos until, no matter what splendid building materials we provide nutritionally, complete confusion reigns in our bodies.

And the innermost, starting with inharmonious thoughts and emotions, becomes the outermost—an inharmonious body. And an inharmonious life.

Thoughts, Feelings and Health

"Worry," one expert has said, "kills more people than cannon"—or, we might add, than germs. It continually sends false alarms, alerts for emergencies and crises that never happen, throughout the entire human system, thus putting all the organs, glands, etc., constantly under stress conditions until the chronic worrier has forced his body to function at four or five times the normal rate.

Is it any wonder the worrier is constantly tired, "nervous," "old before his time"?

Hate and all its cousins set up internal conflicts and tensions so surely that a man you intensely dislike can literally give you "a pain in the neck." Anger wreaks havoc with glands and intestines, drying up digestive juices, so to speak, so that when you eat on an "angry stomach" your food just sits in a lump and you can truly be "fed up" with your fellow man. Digestion and assimilation are disrupted and while your *diet* may be A-plus, your *nutrition* is at zero.

Most psychosomatic symptoms, those traceable to emotional causes, are said to be functional, non-organic. In other words, the organs are not diseased but, under stress and strain, are not functioning properly. However, obviously, continual irritation and malfunction can lead to actual organic damage. And certainly emotional disturbances aggravate organic difficulties. Cardiac patients are advised against excitement, anxiety, and sudden shock. Joe D. Nichols, M.D., of Atlanta, reports that a man he knows who has gout gets along fine "until he gets mad; then he has to go to the hospital."

True, most of us don't go around "worrying ourselves to death" constantly, or flying into a fury every day: But if we indulge in negative thoughts and emotions, and many of us do, we are blocking nature's plans for top physical vitality and efficiency, plus limiting our outlook for a successful life.

Pattern for Positive Living

We have outlined seven rules for positive nutrition.
And seven more for positive health.

Now, let's complete the picture and look at four rules which, coupled with the others, add up to positive living:

One.   *Think* positively.

Two.   *Feel* positively.

Three. *Act* positively.

Four. *Pray* positively.

"Positive," according to Mr. Webster, means: Definitely, explicitly expressed, admitting of no doubt, confident, *affirmative*.

The basis for being able to think, feel, act, and pray, confidently, affirmatively, *positively*, is belief in an all-loving God, a *living*, ever-present God, who made and is part of all things from the blade of grass to the farthest star; and pronounced all that He had made good, *very good*.

Reason tells me this is true. Science affirms it. Intuition tells me it is so. Revelation tells me it is so.

This then, is the base on which I stand when I advocate a confident, affirmative, positive, attitude toward life. From this point of view let's look at the four positive points on our mental and spiritual compass.

Positive thoughts: We are thinking during every waking hour. *What* we are thinking dictates our feelings and actions. Do we accept a false evaluation of ourselves, as worms of the dust, as disintegrating, aging, dying, failing human beings cut off at birth from God and wandering as pilgrims and strangers in an alien world? If we do, we are lying to ourselves. We are taking the negative point of view.

Or do we think of ourselves as immortal, joyous, successful, distributors of an *ever present* Divine Life, Wisdom, and Energy? That is the truth about us. And in the presence of these truthful thoughts we find our sense of inferiority, our fear, our anxieties, and uncertainties, diminished.

Paul Henning, a close friend of ours and one of the great comedy writers of this or any other time, created and then wrote "The Adventures of Bob Collins and Schultzy" for television over a five year period. Paul admitted to Mary and to me that he faced the temptation to negative thinking every single week when he sat down to the typewriter and looked at those sheets and sheets of blank paper. "I sit there and wonder where all the ideas, the scenes, the laughs, the *words* are going to come from to fill them," he confessed. "For an hour or so I even wonder if I'll ever be able to write again, and I fight butterflies under my belt buckle." But Paul never yielded to the temptation to think failure. He met the challenge with positive, confident thoughts and week after week Paul Henning turned out fresh, original scripts, useable largely without a change.

Most of us find we face similar temptations or challenges to think fear, lack, failure and the like, at it isn't the absence of challenge that makes a successful life—rather it is *meeting the challenge with a positive mental attitude.*

We are always talking to ourselves *about* ourselves. And to other people about us. *Don't* let's lie about ourselves *any more.* We are day-dreaming, planning constantly. Are our visions and dreams and plans positive and constructive? Remember, the innermost *does* become the outermost.

It is a Divine law.

I believe with all my heart that I am sort of like a light bulb that burns off the universal dynamo of energy. And so are you. It is all the same Dynamo and the same Light, regardless of our various interpretations of it. It's up to us. We can burn at three watts and be nothing or we can burn at 1,000 and illuminate the world.

And once we take this positive attitude, we have stopped blocking the flow of this power and knowledge and inspiration, and we are cooperating with it instead. When we do this, the wonderful things intended for us from the beginning will crowd into our experience.

Positive emotions: Our feelings will follow our beliefs and thoughts. *If* I believe that it is all the same Dynamo and the same Light, then I must believe that anything I do to help you, helps me. Anything I do to hurt you, hurts me.

There is no such thing as isolation. And if I deceive you, I deceive myself. I believe, no matter how "real" the illusion that we're separated, we *really* are all one.

Understanding, then brotherliness, becomes the affirmative feeling that fills me. Resentment, envy, jealousy, hatred (and with them feelings of inferiority and guilt) are supplanted as *love* takes over.

Christ Jesus instructed us to "love one another," to "forgive one another"—and this was more than ethical teaching. It was a practical approach to positive, good, healthy relationships with each other—and a method for living at peace with ourselves.

Positive actions: are a result of positive emotions and positive thoughts. Our bodily activity responds—and so do our daily affairs. We learn to live and act *now. There is no other time.*

A great burden falls away if we let God run the universe, if we surrender the past and the future into His keeping, and give our full attention to *this day, this minute.*

There's an old saying:

> 'Life is hard,
> By the yard.
> By the inch
> It's a cinch."

The innermost becomes the outermost—if we coordinate our affirmative thoughts and feelings with our action. I think —"I am a happy, joyous, healthful, successful being." I let the thought become a *feeling,* a *conviction.* And now, I *act* as if it were so. I smile. I laugh. I walk and move lightly, effortlessly. Try *smiling* and *acting* your agreement with these positive thoughts and emotions and you'll find, one bright morning that there's no more effort. It is *so.* The natural laws we live under make it so. And you are simply confirming the fact!

It really brings things to a head.

And speaking of bringing to a head in a positive fashion, probably no one in Hollywood has brought more things to a head than the glamorous and versatile columnist, Hedda Hopper. The vegetable and flower arrangements which she wears as hats, for instance, are a positive indication of her very positive nature.

Hedda Hopper can be bawling you out or telling you off but she and her hat will be smiling literally from ear to ear. She is one of the bright spots in any gathering and there is never a dull moment in her very positive presence.

One of the most satisfying results of positive thinking and acting is that it enlarges the horizons of our activity. I remember back when I was at Universal Studios, Henry (Bobby) Costa directed both Deanna Durbin and me in some light, gay and very successful musicals. I was fresh from being "Blade Stanhope Conway" and a "Texan—without—distinction," and marching around singing about vegetables, rah! rah! while Bobby was marching around pooh-poohing positive thinking. He was a mighty good director even then, and was and is, a fine friend. But when Bobby and his lovely wife, Peggy, discovered the positive approach, really began to study and apply it, (they operated) at 1,000,000 horsepower. It was remarkable how his opportunities broadened. Today Henry Costa ranks with the all-time great ones among the Hollywood directors—a man who had the talent and feeling and illumination to give us "The Robe" and "A Man Called Peter."

Positive prayer: Positive prayer is *not* petition or begging. It starts, with me at least, with a kind of adoration and thanksgiving—an awe and wonder at the glory and beauty, the abundance and order of all creation—and a thrill of thanksgiving that I am a part of it. And then follows what Emerson called a "glad conspiring reception, reception that becomes giving in its turn, as the receiver is only the All-Giver in part and in infancy; . . . not exhortation, nor argument becomes our lips but paeans of joy and praise . . . it is God in us which checks the language of petition by a grander thought. In the bottom of the heart it is said: 'I am, by me, O Child! This fair body and world of thine stands and grows. I am; all things are mine; and all mine are thine.' " *

The Fruits of Positive Living

Occasionally, on an interview, I hear a newly orbited Hollywood star say, "I never dreamed any of this would happen to me!"

Don't you believe it!

This is false modesty.

Nobody ever got anywhere without "dreaming it would happen" to them.

The law of positive living is that you cross your bridges before you come to them. You count your chickens before they're hatched. You paint your picture ahead of you with *imagination* (positive thinking) and you back it up with the intensity of belief and desire (positive feeling) plus action (*positive* action) and a receptivity and conviction that you were meant to have beauty and harmony and success. (Positive prayer.)

It also adds up to positive personal charm.

Every person somewhere must make a confession. I am going to confess that I have for many years had a very constant crush on a very lovely lady. I must say that both *her* husband and *my* wife not only haven't objected but actually seem to have encouraged it. This could all sound very serious and very clandestine until I tell you who it is—it is none other than one of the most happily married, perfectly adjusted, wonderfully talented, positive thinkers of all time, My Girl Friend, Dinah Shore (Mrs. George Montgomery).

And, incidentally, my Mary loves her—and George, too.

---

* Emerson's Journal

Things and conditions are solidified dreams and thoughts.

If you are just drifting along, accepting poor health, accepting partial success or failure in any department as "beyond your control," well, you can put a stop to it right now by reversing your pattern. Drop the wishy-washy, negative approach and take a positive stand.

You *can*.

I *did!* And I saw the fruits of it in my own life. And I have seen it in the successful lives around me.

Up the Beverly Hill about a half-mile from the window where I'm sitting someone has just come out into the sunshine on a balcony, someone who is a living proof of this theory. Right now she's doing deep breathing exercises. She does this often. If I put my field glasses on her we can see who it is—Cobina Wright—one of the most gallant creatures ever to inhabit this old planet.

When the crash of 1929 had many of her friends jumping out of windows, Cobina who had lost as much or more than most of them, took a positive stand. All over the country devastated society ladies were wailing, "I've lost everything. I can't go on." But Cobina, with nothing but an awareness and a rich consciousness, said, *"I Can."* And she went on. She probably originated the saying, "Success comes in cans." I've never heard her say "Can't" yet!

My very close friend, Art Linkletter, is a great example of "you are what you think." Art doesn't fall into the trap of false modesty—nor the ditch on the other side, braggadocio. Quite simply, Art just thinks success. He thinks happy talk—and I've never heard him speak against himself, tear himself down, hide behind self-depreciation.

If he hasn't something good to report, he says nothing. And this, to me, is an excellent rule to follow. Art, living it, has not only demonstrated great material success but grandpa Linkletter has an amazing physique and is rarely ill.

Jack Benny has a very positive attitude toward and appreciation for the talents of others. He recognizes, I believe, that it's all the same Light, and anything that benefits another, benefits him. Jack pays his writers more, gets the best technicians, the best costumes, the best people to work on his shows, that it's possible to get. And he doesn't mind a bit having his show stolen (even by a chimp) if it is a *good* show.

Just for the record, Jack is equally positive about money—he just isn't aware of it at all. In reality Benny would give away everything he owned if his wife, Mary, didn't slap his hands.

He has a positive sense that there's success enough to go around—and money enough to go around—and so he shares his star spot and his material wealth—and *there's still all that he could want left over for Jack Benny.*

Almost thirty years ago when Ken Murray was breaking the Palace run, Milton Berle took me (then Blade Stanhope Conway) backstage to his dressing room. Ken, smoking a big cigar, said, "Sit down, pardner." And when I, in my best British accent, said elegantly, "Since I've been in America I'm always delving into personalities and motivation. Could you tell me the motivating factor or rule you go by?" he didn't drop an ash.

"Why, sure, pardner," Ken said. "This is the best rule. In show business there are no rules. And all of them were made to be broken. If it's good, they'll like it. If it isn't, they won't."

Now, restated, that's a very positive rule. It says, and both Ken and I and hundreds of others have proven it, that *you don't copy success.* If you're on the positive team, receptive to positive ideas and inspiration, you'll get fresh inspiration —and there's no limitation imposed on what you can conceive and what you can accomplish.

Frank Tashlin, one of the world's best motion picture directors, a few years ago brought his bride, Mary, to visit us. She seemed like an infant to me and I said, paternally, "What do you want to be?"—biting my tongue just in time to keep from adding, "when you grow up."

Quick as a flash she answered positively, "I am *going* to

be an opera singer." She never let go of that conviction and today she is. The girl's done it. Mary Costa (Tashlin) is known all over the world. London calls her "The world's most beautiful opera singer."

When Doris Day married Marty Melcher, she was a motion picture star—a sort of all-American girl type, supposedly limited to musicals. Together they have put all the *positives to work*, to bring about a solidified dream for Doris. Their own record company, their own music publishing company, their own producing unit. Doris is a singer and a dancer, and a dramatic actress who has been nominated for an Academy Award. They set their vision high and then went confidently toward it. As a couple they have held hands and done it, and I watched them do it.

It works, it really does!

The most dynamic and boldest dreamer I know is Alfred Hitchcock. I have watched him for over twenty years. He would tell me an idea he had and next time I'd see him it would have solidified a little more. Next thing I knew the dream would have become nails, boards, people. A gigantic production underway and then, driving down any street in the world you could see it. The completely solidified dream on the theater marquee, or on a television screen in your own front room. And the more ideas that are solidified, the more he has. *He doesn't run out.* He runs *over!*

Hitch stays right with it. *It never occurs to him that a thing can't be done or that it will be a failure.* And so it has been with his career, and with his personal life—his wonderful wife, Alma, who goes right along with him, his lovely daughter Pat, his grand-children, his beautiful ranch at Santa Cruz.

Lew Wasserman is, today, one of the great success stories of this century. Under Lew, the giant artists' agency, M.C.A., has increased its scope mostly by the potency of Lew's great enthusiasm for everything. You come to Lew with a project and he'll either enthusiastically like it—or enthusiastically turn it down. His decisions are lightning quick and positive. His integrity is unchallengeable. In dealing with artists he's phenomenally sensitive about their feelings, able to absorb them, and *translate them into positive action* in the world of entertainment.

The art of creative or positive imagining is not confined to the world of entertainment, however. I personally have seen the results in the lives of such business men as Henry Kaiser and Conrad Hilton, and such leaders of men as General C. A. Shoop (with his lovely actress-wife Julie Bishop close beside him.)

Someday soon, perhaps, I'll have time to tell, in detail, exactly how this has worked in my own life but for now it is simply a part of the *whole picture of positive living*.

Success is not a destination, but a journey. And an all-round positive attitude governing thoughts and emotions as well as positive health habits are the equipment we need for the journey.

Chapter 15

Making the Most of You

Behind my personal experiments in positive living these past ten years has been a very definite direction.

Acting is an exacting vocation—and my avocation, flying, is exacting as well. Both require physical stamina, energy, quick reactions and sound nerves. Above all, both require organization and expert coordination of body and mind. Body and mind must be sound and clear. And let me say right now that I, personally, have never known a really great actor or actress who was not of sound moral character. Self-discipline as well as looks and talent seem required to get way up to the top—and stay there.

Granted, there are other methods for getting noticed.

I hear that a fish-tailing female attention getter from the movie world, whose talents were never much admired by Ferenc Molnar, rushed up to the playwright, who was seated in a hotel lobby and patted him on the head. It was an attention getting gesture designed to display to the crowded lobby that she and Molnar were friends.

"Please don't pat my head," Molnar said grumpily, "it's the part of my body with which I earn my living. How would you react if someone patted you where you earn yours?"

But the true artists, the great ones of the stage and screen, are highly organized, dedicated individuals rather than sensational personalities.

When I began directing my TV show as well as acting in it, when, over a five year period, we turned out the equivalent of one-third of a feature film every week, I had to be in condition just as surely as a mountain climber or a guy going into the Olympics at Rome.

I found that, almost always, if things went wrong on the set, an emotional upheaval, too much confusion, tension or conflict, it was no use griping about the situation. It wasn't someone else's fault. I had to look for the deficiency in *me*.

"If this is going to come out on schedule," I decided, "I've got to organize Bob, first . . . mentally, emotionally, physically. If the spark plug isn't sparking, well, the engine won't run."

And there was another incentive for my intense training program. In my profession, acting, your living depends on your body, mind, and face. The length of service, all the mastered techniques, all are useful only so long as your body and face are attractive and useful. These must be kept vital if the actor or actress is to go on performing.

This isn't vanity. It's an actor's only inventory.

It's another aspect of the self-discipline the professional entertainer must impose on himself.

And I'd say it is true of every profession, including homemaking—if you want to excel—just as it's true of every man and woman who wants to *enjoy life as long as they live*. I don't think the time ever comes when we don't want to be attractive to other people, to our chosen mate, to the opposite sex, to children, and yes, to animals.

"Everybody wants to be loved," a psychologist friend of mine said the other day. "That's the *great* hunger that has always existed."

Well, the first answer to that is to *be loving* (positive emotion), and the second is to *be lovable* (all the positives including being as attractive as God meant you to be).

"Assembled" Attraction

I thought a long time about the title for this chapter. First I was going to call it, "Re-Building You-As-You-Should-Be." That sounded a little like putting up a concrete wall. Then I thought maybe "Re-Making You-As-You-Should-Be." But I couldn't bring myself to use that because it sounds like direction for what we call, in our trade, the "assembled actor," or the "assembled girl."

A girl shows up at the studio, goes into wardrobe and begins "putting herself together." This is improvement-by-segments-with-artificial-aids. A bra to lift, a girdle to tuck, color on top (applied at home or the beauty salon), make-up to cover, and so it goes.

Or, the "assembled actor" comes on the set in the morning, puts in his teeth, puts in his contact lenses, puts on his toupee, then lifts in the shoes to make him taller, a girdle to make him thinner, shoulder pads for that muscular look. Now he's ready to go out on the set and sing along with a play-back, the sound track made by someone with a fine voice to sing his songs for him.

That is the "assembled actor." And in the past there have been such things. Not many—but a few. Television, however, works at such a pace that there's not time for all that any more.

With the miracle of the camera, the magic that lighting and make-up can do, the illusion is complete for the actor.

But the ordinary person who is held together with elastic, camouflaged by powder, paint, and artificial coloring (and there are such things, too) gets no such breaks.

The attempted illusion is always obviously an attempted illusion.

There is a much better way, nature's way, to make the most of you. And it's never too early or too late to get results.

"Natural" Attraction

This is a true story.

The names and facts have been somewhat changed to keep the wolves away.

A professor in the dental school at a large mid-western university hired an office assistant as an act of Christian charity. They had a common religious affiliation and he knew that her family was destitute.

She was the oldest daughter, an obvious old-maid type, with a sort of ageless oldness about her. Her skin was in a constant state of eruption. Her red hair was dull and stringy. Her figure was flat and colorless. To match all this she had a flat, colorless personality and a positive genius for inefficiency. It was particularly difficult for her to remember simple instructions for five minutes unless she wrote them down —and if she did write them down within five minutes she couldn't remember where she had put her notes.

The professor, while willing to carry his cross, did some moaning about his predicament, and his colleagues, all interested in nutrition, suggested this woman might be a fine human guinea pig for observing the results of improved nutrition.

They recommended not only the Essential Four in her diet, but vitamin and mineral supplements, since it seemed obvious that real deficiencies already existed.

And here's what happened.

Her complexion cleared up. Her stringy red hair took on body and shine and began to grow again. Within eight months her figure had begun to show curves and she was not only getting compliments but wolf calls.

It was noted that she started carrying out instructions more efficiently. In fact, according to the professor, a whole new personality emerged.

Now she wasn't being *assembled* outwardly—but changed

inwardly;—nor was *just nutrition* responsible for the total miracle. As she began to *feel* better, and *look* better, her negative personality was bound to be infiltrated by positiveness, and confidence and joy and these in turn added extra sparkle and vitality to the *total woman*.

When her boss was killed in an accident a year later while she was on a vacation trip there were a dozen M.D.s and dentists who scrambled for her services. And if she is still unmarried it is because she hasn't "chosen" yet. Not because she fails in attraction.

This is the true story of the total rebirth of a woman.

It started with nutrition.

Here are some specific tips for those who want to attain or maintain the original vitality, sparkle, and attractiveness with which nature means to endow us all—fine complexions, glossy hair, alert, sparkling eyes, smooth skin, firm muscle tone.

Glands

Now here we're certainly going to err a little on the side of over-simplification. It isn't necessary to know the exact names, locations, and functions of the eight endocrine glands.

What we do need to know is that they are vital to the health of body and mind and to a balanced personality. The real Master Minds of vitality and well-being, the endocrine glands (and just to show you that I can name them—here they are: pituitary, thyroid, adrenals, pancreas, thymus, pineal, parathyroids, gonads) are the source of the *hormones* which we all know we need but few of us know why. Well, hormone comes from the Greek verb, *hormon,* which means, "I excite." And that is exactly what the various hormones do.

Each of these ductless glands is a complete laboratory making its own magic secretions, or hormones, for controlling bodily activities, or *exciting* our various organs to turn in a maximum performance.

For instance, here is a statement by Dr. Herman H. Rubin, a noted gland specialist, about the pituitary gland: "While the thyroid makes available the supply of crude energy by speeding up cellular processes, the pituitary is responsible for the transformation, expenditure and conversion of that energy into healthful, youthful vitality."

But each and every one of the eight plays an equally vital role. It is a complicated and awe-inspiring miraculous aggregate of action and reaction of such precision and beauty that it's like examining a miniature solar system. And each of these master minds together with their miraculous hormones are interwoven with every secret for youth, beauty, vitality, personality, mental alertness and stability.

These glands must be fed. Without the proper nutritional material they slow down or cease to function. Pep diminishes. Silhouettes get out of hand and we become too fat or too thin. The skin wrinkles and turns sallow. Virility decreases. Baldness sets in.

Now, the beginning of wisdom in *any* beauty or vitality program is to see that the endocrine glands are served.

Do they require some special nutrition?

Not unless a real deficiency exists—in which case your physician is the expert to consult.

But remember, these little dictators are chiefly *protein*. And each and every one of them needs *vitamins* and *minerals* to support efficient action.

This isn't complicated. It isn't confusing. It isn't difficult.

It takes us right back to the Essential Four.

Nature knew what she was doing all along.

Now, let's check some specific areas of physical attraction—for correction and prevention of flaws.

Skin—Smooth, Firm, Youthful

If your skin is sallow, or wrinkled, or crepey, or dry, try some *inner* as well as outer treatment on it.

Accept the fact that your skin is made of protein, and an abundant supply of high-protein foods is the first essential for attractive skin tone.

Your complexion depends on circulation (exercise and deep breathing especially recommended) plus rich red blood —minerals, *iron* and *iodine* (as well as *sulphur*), we remember, plus the *B-complex* vitamins, are our blood bank. And plenty of *gland meats, muscle meats, leafy greens, uncooked wheat germ, milk and cheese, and sea foods* in our diet insure "that school-time complexion."

Small amounts of the unsaturated fatty acids (vitamin F in cold-pressed vegetable oils, such as corn, soy, peanut, etc.) make a valuable *internal* contribution to lovely skin—and olive oil can make a first rate contribution externally in that weekly oil massage.

Vitamin A (found particularly in the deep green leafy vegetables) helps the skin texture and is particularly needed where blackheads, skin roughening and pimples are present.

The youth and beauty *vitamin C* is vital to all cells and tissues, we remember. It gives firmness to flesh and a lack here causes easy bruising as well as the unsightly red splotches often seen on the past-forty skin. *Citrus fruits, raw and canned tomatoes* are the best skin treatment for vitamin C deficiencies.

Now about "wrinkles." A young lady of my acquaintance came home recently and informed her mother that a "charm" teacher in school had said the best way to avoid wrinkles was not to "talk with your face." And I suppose, she would have added, laugh with it, or cry with it, either.

And I recalled a very famous portrait painter who walked up to one of the most gorgeous but unanimated *young* women I have ever seen at a party in the nation's capital and said abruptly (great painters are allowed to be abrupt), "One day, young lady, *if you develop some character lines in your face,* you may be a great beauty."

Now, no one will develop any character lines, nor any

personality, either, if they keep a frozen face for fear of "wrinkles." And if I didn't talk with my face and laugh with it and cry with it, I'd never make a living. The story is told that when a world famous photographer was asked to photograph the world's ten most beautiful women for an international magazine, he wished to include the great Italian actress, Anna Magnani. And Magnani, who is neither young nor orthodox-pretty, agreed to be photographed if the negatives were not retouched. "But I'd just remove a few deep lines," the surprised photographer protested. "You'll do nothing of the sort," Magnani retorted proudly, "I earned every one of them."

But "withering" skin is a different kind of wrinkling from "character lines" and the best way to prevent "withering" is by feeding the skin properly from within.

To sum up—the innermost becomes the outermost, so treat your skin *first* from within—protein, iron, iodine, B-complex, vitamins A and C, vitamin F—or translated into food, plenty of meat, milk, eggs, cheese; an abundance of leafy green vegetables (fresh) and citrus fruits (raw), plus cold pressed oils (or those miraculous seeds, sesame, sunflower, and millet, which contain the B-complex, iron, calcium, as well).

Eyes—Clear and Bright

When I shake your hand and you look me in the eye and say, "I'm fine" I can tell whether you're fibbing or not.

Your eyes are a dead give-away—of fatigue, of where you were last night, of your *true* body age (not the number of candles on your last cake), and of how well you're taking care of that fabulous body the good Lord gave you.

Circles under the eyes *can* come from negative living, but most often they come from negative nutrition, a lack of the iron-rich foods that make good blood.

The Air Force did a good job of making the public aware

of the value of *vitamin A* (yellow and leafy green vegetables—with the publicity emphasis on carrots) in correcting night blindness. But eye fatigue, inflammation, and twitching eyelids also are traceable to this deficiency. A truly serious deficiency can result in "dry eye," a very painful condition where the tear ducts don't supply enough moisture and the appearance is the old "dead-fish-eye" stare, a lusterless, dull, look in either young or old.

Forty-seven adults studied at the University of Georgia suffered twilight blindness when they lacked vitamin B_2. Besides being very sensitive to light, they complained of burning eyeballs, eye fatigue, and a "sandy" feeling under the eyelids. (B-complex foods, Brewer's yeast, wheat germ, and millet, sunflower and sesame seeds can prevent this deficiency from getting a start).

Protein for muscle tone and elasticity, *vitamin C,* which is concentrated in the eye lenses, *Vitamin D, the calcium family* and the *B-complex* group associated with relaxation of nerves and tensions are also needed for attractive, useful, healthy eyes and eyesight. Lack of vitamin B_2, we remember, is definitely related to inflamed eyeballs and eye strain.

Exercise and relaxation of tension in the body generally (remember the Elephant Swing!) are also necessary for eye appeal.

Hair: Glossy, Thick and Your Own!

A woman's hair should be her "crowning glory." Whether it's cut by a mad Italian with pinking shears or is the length of Lady Godiva's, there's no reason why it shouldn't be lustrous and of a pleasing natural hue. And there's no reason why a man's hair shouldn't meet his forehead and still *be his own*.

At least if they both know their nutrition and live it!

Here, healthy hormones from a well-nourished endocrine gland do an amazing job. This calls for, as we've already discussed, plenty of high *protein* and sufficient vitamins and minerals. Lack of *trace minerals* and *iodine,* and *choline* (a substance which is made in our bodies with the aid of certain amino acids that helps keep the fatty cholesterol under control in arteries and liver) have caused the hair on laboratory animals to grow poorly and fall out "in handfuls."

Both our hair and our fingernails are made of *protein* (which can't come as any surprise to you at this point) and both need the particular amino acid found in eggs as well as the high protein foods to be strong and healthy.

Brittle, dry, lusterless hair and, of course the dry, scaly scalp it grows on can be rejuvenated by *vitamin A* (a very busy beauty vitamin!). Vitamin *B-complex, vitamin C,* plus minerals *iron* and *copper* are essential for a clean healthy scalp and a good crop of attractive hair. Sulphur, too, is necessary for hair, nail and skin health—and is supplied by nature in cabbages, Brussels sprouts, and most high protein foods.

How Do You Move and Mend?

You remember the "assembled actor"? How, with the miracle of elastic, make-up, lights, etc., he could give the illusion of youth?

Only one thing betrays him, always.

He *moves* like an "assembled" man. And the "assembled" girl moves like the fraud she is, too. Their muscles and bones give them away. And if our "assembled" actor breaks in any place he mends slowly and badly. And *that* is partially due to lack of calcium.

We need to remind ourselves that "calcium poverty is one common cause of aging that can be corrected."

Calcium and phosphorus (and the sunshine *vitamin D*) are all necessary for "young" bones. If we are "moving old," remember that milk (fresh and dry-powdered), cheese, eggs, lean meat, fish, poultry, and cottage cheese in our diet will keep the supply of calcium and phosphorus coming into the body-laboratory. And watch that the invaluable *vitamin B-*

complex group are included, since these help in the digestion and assimilation of the needed minerals. Add to your diet *vitamin C* (as in citrus fruits) for elasticity and "cement" to hold the proteins all together as well as helping to retain the needed minerals and *proteins,* of course, for muscle tone and replacement material. Then you can move with confidence.

Your well-nourished body won't give the *illusion* of youthfulness, vitality and attractiveness.

It *will be* youthful, vital and attractive!

ᴐᴐᴐᴐᴐ

You and Your Personality

If I'm irritable, quarrelsome, depressed, jittery, or constantly tired I'm aware that I'm not a very lovable character. I'm neither vital nor attractive.

And I've got news for you.

If *you* are irritable, quarrelsome, depressed, jittery, or constantly tired—well, neither are you.

Yet, to suggest that you stop it this instant, that you immediately become positive, serene, gay, energetic, out-going, may be demanding a *physical impossibility*.

It is true that we have to make every effort to think and feel and act positively. But we have to support these efforts by positive eating if we really hope to succeed.

Nutrition does have an effect on the mind and spirit.

And personality "flaws" can stem from "mineral" as well as "moral" deficiencies.

I wish I could pin them all down specifically and say—"for grouchiness eat cottage cheese," or "for laziness take black strap molasses." I've always admired the confidence of the psychiatrist who advertised:

"Positive cure in two years—
Or your mania back."

151

But *good basic nutrition* (the Essential Four) particularly protein, because protein is the builder of all cells that make your nerves, plus these particular tips with which you can safely experiment should give your personality a big lift.

The Nervousness of You

The most common nutritional cause of irritability—when little things bother you out of all proportion, when you are impatient, want to shout back, when other drivers on the road are *excessively* stupid and you want to tell them so, when, as some gals put it, you reach the "I-could-just-*scream*" state of nerves—the probable insufficiency is *calcium*.

And it's a vicious circle. You're short on calcium. Yet constant irritation and constant stress increases the need for calcium. So the more stress and strain and excitement you have—the more you're doing—the more calcium you need. Tests showed that teachers in a California beach city, directing classes, maintaining discipline, use as much calcium as pregnant women during their last months of pregnancy. Obviously the homemaker with a family would use a large amount as well.

Now me, I have three great challenges to irritation. One is the income tax and all the bills. One is directing TV shows on a tight, fast, schedule and the terrific conflict of many volatile personalities in a single operation, and the third is the necessity to keep my own performance as an actor straight through all this. Plus staying awake and productive eighteen hours a day.

Well, I have found the answer for me nutritionally. It's calcium.

Good quality milk and milk products are an excellent source of calcium for bone and teeth. A large percentage of our calcium intake goes to this worthwhile cause. But a tiny, yet vital, percent is used for a very special purpose, for muscle and nerve use and that has to be in a different form called diffusible calcium, or lime.

In nature we're supposed to get this lime chiefly in our drinking water—and in many places, like Texas and Kentucky, where the water filters through limestone, the supply is abundant.

To make sure that I get an adequate supply *I put lime powder* (bought at the drug store—the kind used to make lime water for babies) *in the bottled water I drink at home —and at the studio.* You add a cup of lime water to a gallon of drinking water—and it even makes the water *taste* more refreshing.

Now, of course, as with everything else in the wonderful world of nutrition—*calcium doesn't work alone. Lime water isn't enough.*

In our chapter on minerals (page 76), we discussed the *calcium team,* how the minerals *calcium, phosphorus* and *potassium,* always work together with the vitamin B-complex (one of which, biotin, we've already mentioned as the "cheerful cherub" vitamin) and *vitamins D and F* to calm nerves, strengthen and relax our heart and other muscles, and assist in good quiet sleep that really rests and refreshes.

That's why Catharyn Elwood, in her "lullaby diet" * guaranteed to help "grouchy-in-the-morning-husbands," recommends for the happiest home a steady stream of the whole calcium team—milk, yogurt, skim-milk powder, all dairy products, sun-bathing, wheat germ, Brewer's yeast, liver and leafy greens, fresh vegetables and fruits.

Does it work for the "happy home" department?

Leo Rhodifer, for many years connected with Catharyn Elwood, swears that couples came to consult her who were verging on divorce (irritable, quarrelsome, nervous couples)

---

* *Feel Like a Million,* by Catharyn Elwood—the Devin-Adair Companv. New York, 1955.

who began positive nutrition and the "lullaby diet" and no divorces materialized.

I know that it has worked for me, personally, as a personality stabilizer. The *calcium team* plus the *iron* (the blood bank, remember?) *family group,* since nervousness and lack of confidence are definite symptoms of anemia, are top tips for converting that nervous you into that serene, poised you-that-you-should-be.

By watching these, plus the Essential Four, plus a positive attitude (which you can maintain only if your body permits it) I would say that never, during the five years' course of the Bob Cummings TV Show, no matter how tense and strained things got, did I ever have a real blow up. I may have had a few fake ones (the acting variety) to impress a point on someone in the cast, but it never got under my skin or overworked my glands.

It works for others and it doesn't take a long, long time. I remember the day normally serene and lovely Rosemary De-Camp came to me on the set and said, "I'm so nervous I could just scream. Do you have something for that?"

Well, I gave her some of my supplements that I had at the studio containing calcium and potassium and the other team members for quick action and some advice on lime water and protein (the same that I've just given you) and two days later when I talked to her again she said, "I'm so relaxed—well, everything's just lovely now." So I tried to sell the same idea to "my favorite secretary," Schultzy, but of course happy-go-lucky Ann B. Davis didn't really need it.

But for those of us who do, nature has her own built-in tranquilizers—if we'll just use them.

That Old Tired Feeling

For additional pep, if you really have those lazy bones, and are tired, tired, tired—tired when you go to bed and tired

when you get up—and tired by the least physical exertion—
try more raw foods.

Lysine, one of the *protein components*, is largely destroyed
by cooking, and tests have shown that when human subjects
were deprived of lysine, they tired at the slightest physical
exertion. Lysine helps nutritionally to give us physical
stamina and mental stability.

Many people who suffer from *apathy and lack of get-up-
and-go* are amazed at the new spurt of energy that takes hold
when they start concentrating on proteins, the Essential
Four, going easy on the heavy, starchy, cooked carbohydrates,
and eating plenty of raw foods (including the uncooked protein found in my favorite seeds—one, two, three, repeat after
me—sunflower, millet, sesame!).

One listless lady in her forties who complained that for
five years she had lain in bed very late every morning, although she was awake, because she was just too tired to get
up, really found her personality and entire life altered when
she switched to this New Nutrition.

"I'm practically bouncy," she told me. "I get up early—
look around for things to do. Yesterday I finished some sewing
that's been stashed away for months. I finished the dishes and
housework so early that I went out and vacuumed the car
before lunch. Honestly, I'm having to get used to me. I have
more energy than I know what to do with!"

I hadn't really thought of it this way before but, since I
have been diligently following positive eating and positive
thinking habits, I personally can't remember being tired.

I get bored. I get sleepy. If I'm on a train or a plane and
I have an opportunity to nap, I nap, and I wake up full of
energy. When I wake up in the morning I'm relaxed—I don't
bounce out of bed and hit the other wall—but I'm ready
for the day.

During the day, I just don't "wear out." The moment an
idea comes into my head as to which way I should go—well,
I'm ready. I'm on my way.

And that, to me, is "us-as-we-should-be"—as nature meant us to be, if we adhere to her rules.

Don't Be a Morning Glory

A morning glory, around a race track, is a horse that runs like Man o' War to the first turn and then crosses the wire just ahead of the next race.

Lack of endurance is certainly related to fatigue, but the "morning glory type" usually has big ideas, a big burst of energy and then a collapse before the job is half done.

Extreme laziness of the Ozark Mountain comic type, where Grandma falls in the well and the boys say, "Well, we'll go over in a few days," and then when they find out she doesn't have the energy to crawl out of the well, they find they don't have the energy to pull her out, is great pictorial comedy. But it's a nutritional tragedy, and this condition really exists not only in them thar hills, but all over the nation.

It is said that when these mountain boys aren't leaning against a tree, they're leaning against each other. And that's lack of energy. And that, of course, is nutritional deficiency in a great big way. Not enough proteins. Not enough natural carbohydrates. Not enough minerals and vitamins. But the fast starter who fades fast is a special problem. He's got energy but no endurance.

And here again we are back to the *calcium family*.

The horses in Kentucky are noted for their ability to win. The water in Kentucky is lime-rich.

Race horses that have gotten a bad reputation as back stretch faders have gained endurance plus prize money when diffusible calcium (not a drug but a mineral food) was injected into their muscles before a race.

And people respond just like horses!

The *calcium* team seems not only to calm your nerves, but, in doing so, to release the tensions that wear you out and leave you the stamina you need to finish the day, or the job, or the party, without wilting.

Tips to Top "The Blues"

When we were discussing the B-complex vitamins some chapters back, we mentioned one of them, *niacin,* as the "courage vitamin." A niacin insufficiency, even a reasonably slight one, can affect your personality.

Pellagra, a deadly deficiency disease, formerly prevalent in the south when the diet was basically unbalanced, is known as the "disease of the four Ds" . . . dementia, dermatitis, diarrhea, and finally death.

The people who fall victims to it are normally courageous people, courageous and forward looking. But the first symptoms of the dementia caused by this dietary deficiency are suspicion and confusion. As it progresses, they become discouraged and blue. Next their morale fails. They can't face things. Sometimes, if their outer situation gets too rugged they jump off bridges because they can't stand living in the world. Or they simply leave the world of reality and are confined in institutions.

Dietary insufficiencies can be dangerous, no?

But the point that interests us here is that the subclinical symptoms, suspicion, confusion, lack of morale, the "blues," are quite common psychoneurotic symptoms in places other than the south.

And that where this occurs due to nutritional insufficiencies it can be corrected by a diet high in Brewer's yeast, liver, other meats, dairy products, and good garden vegetables.

The whole vitamin B-complex working together are a great personality pick-up.

The best sources of vitamin B-complex are, once again, *leafy-greens, glandular meats, whole grains and seeds, Brewer's yeast, wheat germ, yogurt;* they are also found in *all meat, fish, fowl, eggs, milk, cheese, green vegetables, legumes, berries, melons, fresh fruit.*

And the richest sources of *niacin* (a member of the B-complex family) are:

FOOD SOURCE	AMOUNT	NIACIN MILLIGRAMS
Barley, whole	½ c.	5.0
Beans, soy, fresh	⅔ c.	4.8
Bran, 100%	½ c.	5.5
Buckwheat, whole	¾ c.	3.0
Chicken, stewed	1 thigh	6.2
Flour, whole peanut	½ c.	19.0
Hamburger	4 oz.	9.2
Liver, beef, raw	2 oz.	15.1
Lobster	3 oz.	5.1
Mushrooms	10 small	6.0
Rice polishings	2 T.	9.6
Steak, beef	4 oz.	8.5
Wheat germ	½ c.	4.8
Yeast, Brewer's	2 T.	10.0
Turkey	100 Gms.	9.8

Now, if you'll just combine imagination with the above information you should be able to come up with a nutritional "pick up" for the "blues" either in salad or one-dish-meal or cocktail form that'll give you a new lease on life.

Once you have supported your efforts at positive thinking with positive eating you'll find a personality emerging that is confident, serene, gay, energetic, and hopeful.

You'll be more attractive than you've ever been in your life.

And you'll know what it's like to *enjoy* each minute of living.

Chapter *17*

࿇࿇࿇࿇࿇

Silhouette Control

American women pay out $300,000,000 annually for foundation garments and girdles "to compress the comestibles," Ernest Blau reports.

And, as I've mentioned, this reporter would estimate from observation in Hollywood, that at least another $100,000,000 must be spent "padding where it ain't."

Yet the solution to both problems is simpler, more permanent, less painful, and absolutely undetectable.

Girth control, whether for the over-weight or the underweight, *starts* with a proper understanding of nutrition. And a pleasing and permanent silhouette is the reward of anyone who will *practice* it.

I know this to be true.

Weight used to be "something to watch" in my life.

But I have not varied more than a pound or two in weight nor an inch or two in measurements since I began to follow the fourteen rules for positive health outlined earlier in this book.

Don't Let It Happen to You

Paulette Goddard once remarked that, if a girl doesn't watch her figure, it's for sure the boys won't. And, say I, vice versa.

But the easiest time to "watch it" is before it's gone.

Living the seven rules for giving the body its needed materials, plus the seven rules for maintaining proper conditions is the best possible guarantee for *preventing* any silhouette problem.

One of those Master Minds, the thyroid gland, is particularly important in silhouette control since a properly functioning thyroid keeps you from becoming either too fat or too thin. A vital hormone, *thyroxine,* is formed when certain amino acids combine with organic iodine in the thyroid gland. To bring adequate building materials to this gland we should provide it with *abundant high grade protein,* plus *iodine* (best sources—sea foods, especially salt water varieties, and plants grown near the sea), plus *thiamin* (vitamin B_1), richly supplied in all gland meats, lean lamb and beef, sunflower seeds and millet, egg yolk, chicken, turkey plus whole grains and fresh fruits and vegetables.

Now I'm often asked—"Just what is the ideal weight for me? I'm five feet, eleven and three quarter inches."

The best weight, I am forced to answer, is the weight at which you *look* and *feel* and *function* best. It varies not only with your height but with the size of your bones and whether your "frame" is large, medium, or small.

Age has nothing to do with it. There is simply no reason for a "middle-aged spread," and health authorities do not view kindly the common supposition that "as you get older you need more padding on your bones."

Here's a basic chart that will help you determine your ideal weight.

Allow one hundred pounds for the first five feet in height, if your frame is "medium" or small, one hundred five pounds if your frame is "large." This you can judge according to your wrist measurement. Then, for each inch over the five feet, add five pounds. If your frame is small you will deduct five pounds. If it is large you will add ten pounds. Here is the way it works chart-wise (with the size of the frame proportionate to the wrist measurement).

WEIGHT SUMMARY TABLE

Measure your height to the nearest 1/4 inch.
Measure your wrist around its largest portion.

Group	Height	Average wrist size	Add for first 5 feet	Add for each added inch	If wrist larger than av.	If wrist smaller than av.	Your ideal weight
1 small	5'0" to 5'3"	5⅝"	100 lbs.	5 lbs.	Add 5 lbs.	Deduct 5 lbs.	
2 medium	5'3" to 5'6"	5¾"	100 lbs.	5 lbs.	Add 5 lbs.	Deduct 5 lbs.	
3 large	5'6" and over	6"	105 lbs.	5 lbs.	If over 6¼" add 10 to 15 lbs.	If under 6" deduct 10 lbs.	

Example: Mary Lou is 5 feet 4 inches tall, and her wrist measures
5 1/3 inches. Since she comes in the "medium" group, you proceed
as follows:

For the first five feet .... 100 lbs.
For each inch over 5 feet .... 20 lbs. (5x4 inches)
Wrist measurement adjustment deduct .... 5 lbs. (less than
average)

Adjusted normal weight .... 115 lbs.

Now, if you are close to your ideal weight—then your silhouette is under control. Don't let it get out of hand. *Take
care of it nutritionally* from now on in the manner outlined
above and you'll have a lovely, lively, attractive silhouette
when you're walkin' your great-grandchildren.

If It's Already Happened

Here are some reducing tips—*do's* and *don'ts.*

And please, from the heart, listen to the *don'ts,* as well as
the *do's.*

Don't take to extremes to reduce.

Don't try to run it off, or melt it off, or rub it off, overnight. There just isn't any way to do it.

Stephanie Redding once wrote of a devotee of the "walk-it-
off" method.

"There once was a lady named Brannagan
Who said, 'I'll be thin if I cannagan.'
So she walked and she walked
Till her weary dogs balked
And she had to sit down on her fannagan."

Don't starve off those extra pounds. You're apt to starve your vitality, and youthfulness, and health right along with them. More than one motion picture star has "blitzed" the weight off repeatedly for pictures only to wind up with a more serious health problem.

This doesn't mean to continue to overload your stomach. It doesn't mean to be careless about carbohydrates. It doesn't mean that you don't have to learn that most difficult exercise of all, leaning against the table and pushing yourself away when you'd dearly love to have seconds—or rich desserts.

It *does* mean that you should and *can* lose weight on an *adequate, proper* diet. But remember, you can be overweight and already half starved nutritionally. And that is partly what this whole book is about—how to be attractive, vital, healthy, (which means in proper focus, pound-wise) at any age, with the aid of positive nutrition.

A really serious weight problem may very well be due to glandular disturbances—that thyroid may not be masterminding as it should. And before you begin any weight reduction, this should be checked with your physician.

But most overweight is *not* glandular. It is *nutritional* and emotional. We'll deal with the nutritional side first.

If you have truly read our fourteen rules for positive health and begun to put them into practice, you should have started to lose weight already. It will come off steadily and surely *as you acquire new food habits*.

And it will stay off.

That is the terrific part of it. The blitz diet or food fad, even when it slices pounds without immediate or dire physical consequences, provides for only *temporary* weight adjustment. The minute you begin to eat again (and you can't keep these odd ball menus up indefinitely) *if you eat according to the same food pattern that got you "out of shape,"* you'll be out of shape and overweight again in no time.

So, if your weight problem is simply a nutritional one (not organic, not emotional) the *first* thing you must do is determine that you are about to embark on a program to re-educate your tastes, and change your eating pattern forever.

The *second* is: make sure that you are getting daily all you *need* nutritionally (even if it's not temporarily all you want). Go back to the Seven Rules for getting proper building material—and be sure you *get* them.

Third: handle your carbohydrates with *extreme* care. Get an abundance of fresh fruits and vegetables to keep up your vitamin and mineral intake using only the low-carbohydrate varieties until you attain your ideal weight.

Fourth: get an abundance of protein—especially the biologically active animal proteins (remember, explorer Stefansson regained and maintained his proper weight on his "Stone Age" meat diet).

Fifth: Remember that you want to be *slim,* but not *scrawny* and that adequate amounts of vitamin F are necessary for lovely, unshrunken skin, real health and calm nerves—so get a small amount of butter, fresh cold-pressed oils, or egg yolk daily.

Sixth: Remember to feed your thyroid its daily needs: *protein, iodine, thiamin.*

Don't count calories. Count food values. Don't eat more than you need. Don't eat one empty carbohydrate. But eat all that your body requires.

If you follow these simple rules with patience you'll have a *new habit of eating and a new silhouette* that will be permanent.

If You Just Can't Win with a Diet

There are those who can accept the above information, and once they understand it, *do* something about it.

But in many instances an "educational program" fails to take root. Mr., and Mrs., and Miss America continue to struggle with the menace of overweight, knowing full well that it robs them of vitality, attraction, *and* endangers their health.

Why?

Here we have to face the emotional side of the problem.

Over-eating or improper eating in the face of the real seriousness of excess poundage is self-destructive just as much, if not as anti-socially, as alcohol or drug addiction.

Nobody wants to be "fat."

It hits our vanity first when we can't get into last year's suit. It hits our pocket book when it interferes with our job. If the condition is organic your physician is the one to help you. But if it is due to over-indulgence then it is a problem of nutrition and a sensible diet plus sensible exercise should be the answer. But too often it isn't.

In the case of the employees at the aircraft factory facing dismissal, we remember a weight control clinic was set up to meet each week for sixteen weeks. A diet, advice, warnings, all were provided. The rest was up to the individual. Yet after two weeks the women ceased losing weight. They could not stay on their diets. They had become compulsive eaters and their will power seemed insufficient to help them help themselves.

Again why?

Because the difficulty was primarily in their emotional nature. Eating releases tensions. It can be caused by sexual problems, lack of affection, emotional upheaval such as sorrow or loneliness, or it can be simply a method of escape. Here the mind and feelings, not the mouth, cause the extra weight. Yet, while physical hunger can be appeased with an apple or a glass of milk (or a banana split, although I don't recommend it!) spiritual hunger has never been assuaged with food yet! What, then, can be done?

We come now to combining positive eating with positive thoughts, emotions, and actions. And, when we *engage the whole person,* it works. Boy, does it work! I heard with great interest the experiences of a nutritionist who made this discovery for herself. She had been going through a period of emotional tension and insidiously, pound by pound, had gained too much weight. She was faced with having to reduce and she'd found that she couldn't do it. For two days she would stick to her diet and then she'd fall for a slice of banana cream pie. "I was ashamed and miserable for I began to see that theory and practice were two different things," she admitted. Something more was needed here. She remembered how many times she had compared compulsive eating to compulsive drinking and that seemingly incurable alcoholics had found release in Alcoholics Anonymous by asking a Power greater than themselves to help with their problems.

During the next ten weeks, according to her report, she lost a pound a week. It was a pleasant and effortless, as well as highly rewarding experience, she said. Here is the pattern she followed for loss of weight. "As an individual," she said, "I can assure you that it worked for me. As a nutritionist I know it can work for anyone."

1. Take a definite, positive, stand. "I will lose weight!"

2. See your family physician for a check-up. (He will locate possible organic causes and advise you how much weight you need to lose.)

3. Attain a sound, well-balanced reducing diet either from your physician or a reliable nutrition authority. (There is no safe quick-reducing scheme and, if there were, the benefits would not last unless the tensions were relieved and a sounder, permanent eating-pattern developed.)

4. Set up a regular pattern of eating, whether it is three meals a day or six (if the latter, of course you do not increase the total amount of food recommended in the diet.) Acknowledge God's presence in the form of your own choosing before each meal.

5. Evaluate the tensions which are causing you to over-eat. Know that you will have God's help in eliminating them.

6. Accept the fact that this will mean a new way of life both spiritually and nutritionally, not just for now, *but for always*. Surrendering your tensions to God instead of placating them with cream puffs is bound to have an all-round effect on your daily life.

7. Have set times for spiritual reading, for meditation, for recharging your dynamo, but keep in mind round the clock that God is there for your comfort and support and that no problem is too small for His attention. (Meditation and an awareness that God is within you is the sound way to feed those spiritual lacks that calories can never feed.)

8. Remember that the body was meant for use. Use it. Keep it fit. Setting up exercises each day (preferably in the morning) stimulate circulation and firm muscles. Half an hour evening walk (it isn't the speed but the time that counts) will do wonders for relaxing the body before bed-time.

9. Weigh yourself once a week always at the same time, wearing the same clothes. Be grateful to see a pound disappear.

10. Take the long viewpoint. You didn't accumulate this surplus weight in a week. You won't lose it in a week either.

11. Relying on God you can keep your attitude calm and cheerful. Don't discuss dieting with your friends as if it was a cross too great to be borne. Actually, staying on this spiritual and physical diet one day at a time is a great spirit lifter. You'll find it dissolves a lot of guilt complexes.

12. Know firmly and with conviction that, with God's help, you can achieve your goal!

~~~~~~

Chapter 18

Sex and Salad

There's a story told in nutrition circles about a bride who had been advised by a well meaning friend that sea food would give her husband that extra oomph a honeymoon demands. So she went into a fish stall to buy some oysters.

"Large or small, ma'am?" she was asked.

"I really don't know," she stammered. "They're for a man with a size 16½ collar."

But the real joke is that here, at least, nutrition has been given consideration throughout the ages. Some of the concepts, however, were pretty weird. For instance, Madame de Pompadour, one of history's most celebrated courtesans, whose position at the court of Louis XV depended largely on a warm nature and sustained physical charm, was given to bolstering both with exotic diets. For breakfast she drank truffle and celery soup washed down by hot chocolate which had been laced with triple vanilla and ambergris.

Now, nutritionally speaking, this is neither very potent nor very wise.

But vibrant physical attraction plus the ability to enjoy a long, normal, healthy, sex life *is* based on normal healthy glands. And the first requisite for these is proper nutrition.

The glands that play the major role in this picture are the thyroid (the pace-setting gland that we discussed in relationship to silhouette control) and the gonads (*ovaries* in women, *testes* in men).

If the thyroid slows down, sexual powers are decreased. And if the gonads are not provided with proper building materials, the invaluable hormones it is their function to produce are in short supply.

The first building material necessary is *protein*.

In an experiment a group of normal males were placed on a low protein, high carbohydrate, diet. The result was a definite loss of interest in the opposite sex.

We already know that the thyroid, to set a proper pace, must not only have *proteins,* but *iodine* and *thiamin* (vitamin B₁). And for healthy sex glands not only *protein,* but *iron* and *copper* (which we know works with iron) are essential.

Vitamins also play their role in this vitality act.

To reinforce the functioning of the sex glands, to keep all the mucous membranes of the body in good condition, *vitamin A* and *vitamin C* are needed.

To keep the pituitary gland producing the hormones which stimulate the sex glands and prevent a decrease in sexual desire, we need our friend *Thiamin* (vitamin B₁).

The sunshine *vitamin D* works with the sex hormones to increase sexual desire, and *vitamin E* keeps the sex glands in good condition and has to do with fertility.

Proteins we've discussed—and discussed. And the foods containing the richest sources are listed on page 64. Remember that some of the amino acids do not survive cooking *so be sure to get some raw protein daily* (as in sunflower, sesame, millet seeds, nuts, and fruits and vegetables).

Now here is a review of the other building materials necessary to keep your physical vitality and attraction lively and lovely.

IRON	COPPER	VITAMIN A
Liver	Molasses	Deep green vegetables
Tongue	Liver	Liver
Heart	Leafy greens	Egg yolk
Muscle meats	Berries	Cheese
Molasses	Whole grains	Whole milk
Peanuts	Oysters	Butter

Apricots
Wheat germ (uncooked)
Leafy greens
Fresh fruits
Lima beans
Kidney beans
Peaches

Clams
Egg yolk
Dried fruits
   (esp. apricots
    and figs)

Green vegetables
Yellow vegetables
   (esp. carrots)
Yellow fruits
Sunflower seeds

THIAMIN
(Vitamin B₁)

Wheat germ (oil or
   uncooked)
Whole wheat flour
Brewer's yeast
Oysters
Milk
Liver
Gland meats
Lean lamb & beef
Chicken
Egg yolk
Sunflower seeds
Millet
Sesame seeds
Fresh fruits
Vegetables
Leafy greens

VITAMIN D
(sunshine)

Egg yolk
Milk
Oysters
Fatty fish
Tuna
Salmon
Sardines

VITAMIN C

Citrus fruits
Tomatoes
Fresh vegetables
Melons
Apricots
Strawberries
Leafy greens

VITAMIN E

Cold-pressed veg. oil
   (wheat germ, olive,
    corn, soy, etc.)
Sweet potatoes
Liver
Oat meal
Brown rice
Turnip greens
Eggs
Fish
Sardines
Barley

Lelord Kordell, in *Eat and Grow Younger,** says, "Hundreds of cases of so-called 'impotency' in men and 'frigidity' in women, have responded to diets purposely planned to provide generous amounts of foods rich in high proteins, iron and copper, and vitamins A, D, E, and thiamin."

With the charts listed above and a little creativity and imagination you should be able to come up with a really Potent Pompadour Cocktail.

Or a really Scintillating Salad.

Salad for Sex and Sparkle

Let's see now what we can do with a little creative imagination plus the Key Chart (pages 106-107) in bringing to-

---

* *Eat and Grow Younger*, by Lelord Kordell, The World Publishing Company, Copyright 1952.

gether in one meal a luncheon menu that will guarantee long life to those endocrine glands that in return give us life-long sexual vibrancy.

VEGETABLES—LEAFY GREEN	FISH (salt water especially)	SHELL FISH
High protein	*High protein*	*High protein*
Natural carbohydrate	*Iodine*	*Iodine*
Vitamin A	Sulphur	Sulphur
Vitamin C		
Vitamin E	*Special values*	
B-complex (includes thiamin)	Sardines Vit. D&E	
Calcium	Tuna Vit. D	
Phosphorus	Salmon Vit. D	
Potassium		
Magnesium		
Iron		
Copper		
Sodium		
Chlorine		
Trace minerals		

EGGS	NATURAL VEGETABLE OILS (Cold-pressed)
High protein	*Vitamin E*
Vitamin A	*Vitamin F*
Vitamin D	
Vitamin E	
Vitamin U	
B-complex (including thiamin)	
Phosphorus	
Magnesium	
Iron	
Copper	
Trace Minerals	

FRUITS	TOMATOES—CITRUS FRUITS RAW CABBAGE
Incomplete *protein*	*Excellent source Vit. C*
Good carbohydrate	Incomplete protein
Vitamin A	*Vitamin A*
Vitamin C	Vitamin P
B-complex	*B-complex*
Iron	Chlorine

Phosphorus
Potassium

Special values

Grapes	Vit. P
Prunes	" P
Plums	" P
Peaches	Iodine
Bananas	Iodine
Dried apricots	*Copper*
Dried figs	"
Cherries	Vit. P
Cherries	Iodine
Apricots	Vit. P
Apricots	*Iron*
Apples	Vit. P
Apples	Iodine

Zinc
Cobalt
Calcium
Phosphorus
Iron
Sodium
Potassium
Trace minerals

Special values

Cabbage juice—Vit. U
Cabbage   sulphur

NUTS

High *protein*
Calcium
Phosphorus
Iron
Sodium
Potassium
Magnesium
Trace minerals
Vitamin F

Unblanched almonds	*Peanuts*
Good protein	*Good protein*
B-complex	*B-complex*

Thiamin (a member of the B-complex family) is a water soluble vitamin that is partially destroyed in cooking, so the salad technique can be most effective here as well as providing us with some of the amino acids which heat destroys.

Now, combine a sea food salad—tuna, salmon, with a hard cooked egg and plenty of leafy greens (mix up your lettuce—head lettuce isn't the *only* one nature thoughtfully provided for you—and remember water cress, parsley, and tender young spinach leaves add food value as well as flavor and eye appeal). Garnish with tomato and you've got a really sparkling creation that will change your life.

Or try a fresh fruit salad on a bed of leafy greens and sprinkle some chopped nut meats (or the magic sesame or sunflower seeds) over it. And once again you've come up with a real treat for the glands that will bring you sparkle and sex appeal.

Don't forget that there are exciting nutritious salad dressings that add to your menus both for fruit and vegetable salads. They use those cold-pressed oils that contain invaluable vitamin E and I've suggested one that uses a raw egg yolk—again providing thiamin and the amino acids without risking their loss in cooking.

FRENCH DRESSING *(Basic)—about ½ cupful*

Combine:
    ¼ teaspoon salt
    ¼ teaspoon paprika
    1 tablespoon cold-pressed oil
    1 tablespoon vinegar or lemon juice
    ¼ teaspoon dry mustard
    1 teaspoon sugar

Beat these ingredients well until they are smooth.

Add:
    2 tablespoons olive oil

Beat again. Add:
    1 tablespoon vinegar or lemon juice
    3 tablespoons olive oil

Peel and add:
    1 clove garlic

To this basic dressing you can add:
    chopped parsley, or
    chives, or
    other herbs.

CHIFFONADE DRESSING—about 1½ cupfuls—excellent on a mixed green or sea food salad

Prepare:
    ½ cup French dressing

Add to it:
    2 chopped hard-cooked eggs
    2 tablespoons chopped pepper

2 tablespoons chopped parsley
2 teaspoons chopped chives
1 teaspoon chopped onion

NUT DRESSING—about ½ cupful

Pound to a paste:
    2 tablespoons pecan nut meats
    2 tablespoons blanched almonds

Beat in:
    ¼ cup lemon juice
    ¼ cup olive oil
    ¾ teaspoon salt
    ¾ teaspoon paprika

EGG YOLK DRESSING

Peel, then mince fine:
    4 garlic clove sections

Beat in:
    1 egg yolk
    ½ teaspoon salt

Add slowly, beating constantly:
    1 cup oil

When dressing thickens, beat in:
    ½ teaspoon cold water
    1 teaspoon lemon juice

If the dressing is not thick enough, beat an egg yolk and add the dressing to it very slowly, beating constantly.

Madame Pompadour, with her limited knowledge and her vanilla and ambergris in hot chocolate and her truffles, only succeeded in gaining too much weight and died when she was a little past forty. Any man or woman today who will *use* the knowledge modern nutrition has provided can stay slim and physically vibrant during a long and healthy life.

Chapter 19

The Time
of Your Life

As Americans, according to Dr. Stanley M. Garn, we may be *"eating our way to the cemetery beginning in the perambulator."*

Dr. Garn, of Antioch College, an authority on physical growth, expressed this concern, particularly about teen-agers, in a volume on "The Nation's Children," a publication prepared for the White House Conference on Children and Youth.

"Reviewing the dietaries of some of our teen-agers," he wrote, "I am struck by the resemblance to the diet that Dr. Olaf Nickelsen uses to create obesity in rats . . . (which) may be . . . good for the undertaker and bad for the populace."

Fred D. Miller, D.D.S., feels that the college youths who adhere to a frivolous diet (one pretty well devoid of food values and catering merely to pleasure tastes) "pay through the teeth." But this leading dental-nutrition pioneer adds that it isn't only the "kids." Remember that our teeth are a very good indication of our general nutritional health and then consider Dr. Miller's comment. "What are the conditions in the mouths of *adult Americans* today?" he asks. "First, so many men are being rejected from the army because of bad teeth that they are not only the highest single cause for rejections (nearly a fourth of all rejections according to the last statistics I have seen) but an indication of disaster ahead unless something drastic is accomplished. When you stop to consider the age of these draftees and the army's low requirements, you get some idea of the appalling dental health of under-middle-aged American men.

"Second, the average American loses *all* his teeth at forty-nine and has full upper and lower dentures (false teeth to you) made."

Dr. Miller then states flatly—"*Tooth decay is not normal. Tooth decay is a sign of illness*" . . . and that this "illness" which he blames on improper nutrition, will surely show up in other parts of the body if we continue "the kind of dietary abuses that eat holes in tooth enamel."

Now, all that is very sad, a negative, even shocking picture. But here's the good news. While you're *never too young* to start benefiting from the fourteen rules for positive health, you're *never too old,* either. Whatever your age is right this minute, is the right time of your life to bring the benefits of positive living into your actual experience.

But each age group faces special problems. Let's see what they are and what can be done about them.

Teen-Age Mirror

Our schools, from first grade on, are doing their level best to educate our children to an understanding of proper nutrition and the need to *live* it.

But somehow there's a gap between theory and practice.

I think maybe some of our teen-agers have gotten confused by the long technical terms and don't really understand that the lessons are about them and their insides, like the girl who was asked to tell what the blood does and wrote: "The blood flows through the elementary canal into the abominable canopy. It is also putrified in the lungs by inspired air. The heart beats and stirs up the blood and digests the food." If she can't tell what's wrong with *that* picture, she's apt, one day soon, not to be breathing at all.

And some have understood all right but haven't made the connection between getting an A or B in Home Economics or Biology and *doing* the things they learn. Parents tend to leave them more on their own and if their nutrition facts are all on ice in some note book they can still wind up like Miss Perkins (who quite probably got an A in biology, too). Anyhow, as an example, meet Miss Perkins:

> "There was a young lady named Perkins,
> Who simply doted on gherkins,
> *In spite of advice,*
> She ate so much spice,
> That she pickled her internal workin's."

The italics, as the experts say, are *ours* but the theme is obvious.

A friend of mine who is a public servant in the nutrition field told me of instances where high school principals in good economic areas (which just means 'no excuse' neighborhoods) were very concerned about the signs of poor nutrition in teen-age students—not only skin-figure-dental-wise, but in listlessness, poor concentration and work far below capacity. They were eating plenty—of the wrong things. In some instances they were not C or D students, they were just overstuffed and underfed!

"I've interviewed thousands of teen-agers, visited their homes, good homes, in good neighborhoods," she told me. "There seem to be three major problems—the 'no-breakfast' habit—eating-on-the-run even at home—and snacks, which fall into the problem class only because of their selection. Pinned down, most of them *know* what to eat, and when, they just don't *do* it!"

A group of teen-agers who examined this problem themselves added two items to this list—lack of nourishing lunches, either bought or packed—and girls following foolish fad diets.

The vital seriousness of The Case of Mal-nourished Teen-agers was brought to light at a National Food Conference in Washington in 1958, and leaders of the food industries were shocked into more than criticism. They acted. Beginning in September, 1959, a nationwide service was launched to focus the attention of teen-agers on their eating habits not only through schools but through youth groups. And the results have shown that there's nothing apathetic about this group once they've been shown something amiss and given a chance to start correcting it.

A Youthpower movement entirely composed of teen-agers has orbited as a result of this new service. Their slogan is Food Comes First, and they've been very enthusiastic about launching such things as editorial and poster contests to prove it. In February, 1960, one hundred and sixty-five members of the Youth power movement rallied at their First Annual Congress in Chicago.

First they had a good old gripe session.

That, to me, is healthy America!

"What is the trouble? Where is it?" they demanded of themselves. "Let's face facts."

They discussed eating-on-the-run, the no-breakfasts and empty-calorie-snack habits, as well as foolish dieting. They were pretty frank about the causes and parental shortcomings in these departments didn't escape observation even if they escaped blame.

How could they?

These Future Mothers and Fathers of America had to know the dangers and mistakes before they started running homes of their own. No breakfasts and eating-on-the-run got some wistful comments about the need for Family Meals. Many of those who had studied home economics or Scout cooking courses thought home meals were poorly balanced (and we won't go into what *that* means again!—like well balanced means meat, milk, greens, fruits—right?) and several of the boys referred to usual lunch spots (and even some cafeterias) as Ptomaine Palaces. But by and large, they were all willing to concede that as teen-agers, they should be able to help correct most of these conditions if they were more selective when eating out and tactful with Mom at home about offering to help with new meal planning and cooking. But they did need parental help and adult guidance.

On the Snack Score they felt that these habits were chiefly a "pack complex," that they ate when and what- and where- "the crowd eats." Now here's a theory that should be interesting to all mothers, present and future, which is that as a nation *we teach our young to place undue emphasis on sweets,* especially by using them as treats, rewards, sources of comfort, or withholding them as punishments. Take a young mother I once knew who wouldn't give her small daughter sweets just before dinner, but five minutes later, when the little girl fell off her tricycle and came howling through the door, mamma comforted her with candy.

Here it's a good thing to remind ourselves that, while physical hunger can be appeased with food, food simply doesn't truly meet our social, and emotional needs.

The Youthpower Congress recognized these problems and they got down to what can be done to answer them. When you look at their conclusions you can't call these young people "soft" or uninterested in positive living. They decided:

To ask parents and teachers to help them improve school and family meals.

To break the "pack complex" by being leaders and not sheep, by setting an example on healthful snacks and packed lunches, spreading information by editorials and personal enthusiasm about breakfast and lunch needs, and the dangers of fad diets.

Above all, to try and institute, or re-institute, dinner as the Happy Family Occasion of the day. I think this H.F.O. is a terrific idea, myself. Mrs. Harry Michaelson, director of the Children's Department, American Institute of Family Relations believes: *"The last stronghold of family unity is the dinner hour."* Them's big words, too!

If you're willing to be the Joan of Arc of the Family Dinner Table here are a few tips Mrs. Michaelson adds to those we've already rehearsed on good nutrition.

Don't make food and table manners the focal point of conversation.

Don't gear your talk to the youngest. (Baby's babble doesn't need a response beyond a kind smile.)

Don't let it become a gripe session. (Where's the unity, if you fight your way through the meal?)

Do sit down and stay down. (Letting everybody run to the kitchen for forgotten items still makes it eating-on-the-run. Do the thinking for the whole meal ahead of time!)

Do give everyone a chance in the conversation. (When in doubt try word games, or general topics like sports and school. This will increase social awareness, too! And baby can babble his opinions in unchallenged peace!)

And do say Grace before the meal begins. I personally am all for this. But this isn't *only* a personal or religious idea. It's sound psychology and good nutrition. The age-old custom of grace before meals has the endorsement of modern science for physical as well as ethical reasons. Eating as a reverent act (to supply that "temple of God," remember?) following sincere family worship, is apt to preclude "wolfing" or quarreling, both enemies of sound digestion. And to put real steel girders in this "stronghold of family unity" what better way than to remember that "The Family That Prays Together Stays Together"?

That is a positive plank in the platform of positive living.

The Young Adult

We usually think of the young adult as being at the prime of physical well-being—and it is true that generally speaking this is the age at which the average American *feels* the best. The physical stress and emotional strain of adolescence is behind. The "childhood diseases" have been weathered. And any flaw which is developing from dietary deficiency has rarely made a firm enough inroad to show marked outer effects.

Yet we have already, in an earlier chapter, reviewed the over-all picture of health in the young men of draft age and found it deteriorating in contrast to a similar draft thirty-two years previous.

And I read the following article in "The Insider's Newsletter," New York, February, 1960,*

"HEART TROUBLE—FOR THE YOUNG. The Armed Forces Institute in Washington reports an alarming increase in heart cases among young American males. Studying the autopsies performed on 389 pilots killed in air accidents, the Institute found: Seventy percent of those in the 20 to 24 age group had some hardening of the coronary arteries. Fourteen per cent had marked hardening. In pilots 30 to 34, 79 percent had the same trouble—and 32 percent had it seriously.

"The same percentages hold true for flyers or non-flyers, the Institute has found. Possible explanation: lack of proper exercise in modern life; too much fat in our diets."

Nobody, neither experts nor laymen, seems to doubt that poor nutrition coupled with violations of our other rules for positive health are a prime factor here.

Yet it is difficult to make the young adult face the seriousness of the situation for two reasons. First, he or she probably notices as yet few of the outward symptoms of fatigue, wilting appearance, low resistance, that they are constantly courting. And second, the young adults are primarily concerned with making a place for themselves in a highly competitive society, or making a home for their children—and they feel they just *don't have time to take care of themselves.*

---

* "The Insider's Newsletter," copyright 1960 by Cowles Magazine, Inc.

I went through that stage myself and I know what a busy time it is.

I remember a young mother I knew back in those days, the wife of another struggling young actor, who wore herself to a frazzle keeping a lovely little home and taking first rate care of three babies. Those babies were never without their vitamins, their minerals, their strained, scraped, puréed foods. They were really Bouncing Babies—the perfect products of perfect nutrition. And then one day mamma collapsed in the kitchen and was taken to the hospital. The diagnosis was *mal-nutrition.*

She simply "hadn't had time" to care for mamma.

And when mamma collapsed, the family collapsed as well.

The same thing applies to the young man who's "too busy making his mark" to abide by nature's simple rules for health. The very finest young constitution can be undermined by lack of sleep, too much tension, too little and improper nourishment, too many stimulants to try to fill the gap, until, just as the hard work begins to pay off, just as the mark is hit, the body rebels.

The young adult *truly* doesn't have time to neglect the body.

They don't have the *right* if they have dependents or talents, or hope to bear healthy children, or insure a bright future, to abuse, starve, or maltreat the instrument which must carry them to their goal.

And honestly, the more ambitious the young adult is the more quickly he or she will realize that they *can't afford* to lose one bit of the health, vitality, mental alertness and physical attraction that they will need to run a good race, fight a good fight—and be able to fully enjoy the victory.

The Challenge of Middle Life

It is reported that a lady trying to strike up a conversation with the caustic-tongued George Bernard Shaw, made the sprightly observation that youth is a wonderful time of life.

To which GBS replied, "Yes. Too bad it's wasted on the young."

By the time most of us arrive at middle life we are readily aware that, to keep our youthful enthusiasms and vigor, we had better "take care of ourselves." It is in middle life that the exercise machines, the rejuvenation creams, the paint pots and dyes, begin to get a big focus for those fading forties and fast folding fifties.

But our real accent should be on our rules for positive living because nature is the most generous of all law makers. The minute we begin to obey her, regardless of past violations, we can get beneficial results. I know this for a fact because I was forty years old before I adopted and began really to *live* all fourteen of our rules for positive health.

It's true that I hadn't committed any violent abuses of nature's laws or run into any organic difficulties. No, I'd just been fumbling around in the wonderful wonderland of nutrition. But John D. Rockefeller was in his late sixties, and a man who had never had a robust constitution, when some obscure digestive troubles reduced him to extreme weakness and almost to death.

At that point he began strict adherence to a prescribed diet and other health measures—whereupon he out-lived two of his physicians and reached the age of 97 years and ten months —a long and useful life.

Now, all the rules for rejuvenation nature's way have been covered. But to give you some further encouragement here are a few words of advice from people who have proved that it is effective.

The first list comes from that baseball wonder, Leroy Satchel Paige. Nobody knows exactly how old Satchel Paige is, nor exactly how long he has been pitching, nor exactly how long he will continue to pitch. But Satch has been around a long, long time. And here is his advice on:

How to Stay Young

"Avoid fried meats which angry up the blood.

"If your stomach disputes you, lie down and pacify it with cool thoughts.

"Keep the juices flowing by jangling around gently as you move.

"Go very lightly on the vices such as carrying on in society. The social ramble ain't restful.

"Avoid running at all times.

"Don't look back. Something might be gaining on you."

And not long ago an observant female sports fan, Mrs. Barbara Greppin, of Rochester, New York, wrote *This Week* Magazine, asking, "I've noticed that many of our sports champions are middle-aged, yet still at their peak. What's their secret?"

A roving editor went forth to interview such sports greats as Slammin' Sammy Snead, 47, who had just finished the best year of his career; Ted Williams, who, in his 41st year, tied with Mel Ott for third in the all time home-run-hitters, had a batting average of 316, with 98 hits, 15 doubles, and 29 home runs; Gardnar Mulloy, the tennis star who, at 40, was ranked number one in the United States and at 46 was still a doubles ace; boxer Archie Moore (who sometimes claims to be 53); A. D. Beveridge, 44-year-old captain of the U.S. Championship polo team; and the like.

Editor Leslie Lieber summed up his report, "How Champions Stay Young," * thus:

"1. Don't stop exercising in middle age.

2. Get at least eight hours sleep a night. If your body requires it, take a nap during the day.

* "How Champions Stay Young," by Leslie Lieber. *This Week* Magazine— July 5, 1959.

3. Eat a solid high-protein diet rich in beef, eggs, vegetables, and salads. Drink adequate quantities of milk and cut down on rich desserts.

4. Vitamin and food supplements? Well, at least 95 percent of the antique athletes we talked to swore by them. They're a basic plank in the health platform. See your doctor for what kind."

So you see, it works. It really does. Don't give up. Don't consent to wilt or fade! *You don't have to.* Good nutrition plus sound health rules can put you and keep you in top form at *this time of your life,* if you start today and stick with it.

Chapter 20

How to Live Long — And Love It!

Since I haven't yet reached the Golden Age, that of Senior Citizen, I now have to go beyond my personal experience, but of one thing I am convinced.

The rank of Senior Citizen should be a proud and respected one, and the life of a Senior Citizen should be both happy and useful . . . not a fearful, anxious approach to the scrap heap.

I feel sure Harry Emerson Fosdick, the inspiring eighty-two-year-old clergyman, is right when he says, "It is magnificent to grow old, if one keeps young," and the best method of attaining a long, pleasurable life was well expressed by Herbert Spencer when he wrote, "The whole secret of prolonging one's life consists in doing nothing to shorten it."

Nutrition-wise we've covered the ground already on "how to" start now doing nothing to shorten it. And now here are a few health tips for those who have already arrived at the Golden Age.

Dr. Henry C. Sherman, noted bio-chemist of Columbia University, believes that the prime period of human life could be extended by a moderate increase in calcium in the diet of those in or approaching the ranks of Senior Citizens,

plus eating twice the minimum amount of protein, and a
sizeable increase in the daily intake of Vitamins A and C.

Dr. Sherman arrived at this conclusion as a result of studies
conducted on albino rats (whose chemistry is similar to that
of human beings) and translates into this practical buying
key: one-fifth of the food budget on milk and cream; one-
fifth on fresh fruits and green vegetables; three-fifths on
meat, eggs, fish, enriched or whole grain cereals and breads,
nuts, and butter.

Life insurance statistics prove conclusively that too much
weight is a hindrance to a long and healthy Golden Age.
When in excess of the body's needs, fat is, in all of us, an
obstruction in the placement and action of the organs, a dead
weight to haul around, and the cause of additional miles of
blood vessels which put added strain on the heart. So we
can see the good sense in the advice given by the famous
English physician, Sir William Osler, that after fifty, every
man should begin to modify his diet.

This is the impersonal advice of the modern experts after
examining laboratory experiments, vital statistics, and case
histories. But to me one of the greatest, most interesting and
most inspirational authorities who ever dealt with this subject
was a Venetian nobleman living in the middle of the fifteenth
century, who *lived* one of the most remarkable and successful
experiments of all time. He wrote four discourses which were
published first in English as: *"A Sure and Certain Method
for Attaining a Long and Healthy Life."*

Luigi Cornaro, born of a noble and wealthy Italian household in the middle of the 1400's, was a physical wreck facing
invalidism and death at the age of thirty-six and a healthy,
happy, useful man in full possession of his faculties at a hundred and three.

The "miracle" of how the transformation was wrought
which brought Cornaro, a young man of naturally weak constitution who had undermined it almost totally by dissipation
before the age of forty, to Cornaro, who spent sixty-three

more glowing, vigorous years living the life of man-as-man-should-be, in health and buoyancy of spirit, is the subject of his treatise.

And his "Sure and Certain Method" on "The Art of Living Long," as he describes it in the four discourses, the first written at eighty-three, the second at eighty-six, the third at ninety-one, and the last at ninety-five, is, quite simply, a description of the life of Moderation.

Cornaro was "reborn" in health and mental attitude when he became a devotee of diet, personal hygiene, and a positive common sense approach to life. Physically he guarded against excesses, including those of extreme heat, cold, and fatigue. He allowed nothing to interfere with his sleep and rest periods. An ill-ventilated room he would not tolerate. An excess of sun and wind he considered unwise. He believed that *"not to satiate oneself with food is the science of health,"* and he was extremely careful in the selection of what he ate—mainly bread (undoubtedly whole grain in the fifteenth century), bread soup, eggs, meat (veal, kid and mutton were the most readily available), poultry and fish.

"All persons," Cornaro insists, "should observe the temperate life prescribed as nature's highest law."

Nor did he confine his attention strictly to rules for the physical man. Far in advance of his time he recognized the influence of the mind and emotions, and gave a fine prescription for immunity from psychosomatic symptoms.

"I have also," he wrote, "preserved myself, as far as I have been able, from those other disorders from which it is more difficult to be exempt; I mean melancholy, hatred, and the other passions of the soul, which all appear greatly to affect the body."

In a testimonial written during Cornaro's lifetime by Hieronimo Gualdo (circa 1560) we have an on-the-spot-report of the life of this remarkable man.

"In a word, from a despairing and almost helpless invalid unfit for either work or enjoyment, he (Cornaro) became not only a man of perfect health, singularly active and happy, but also such an example of self-restraint as to be the wonder and admiration of all who knew him, earning and receiving the title of *THE TEMPERATE*. The mildness and sweetness of his altered disposition at the same time gained for him the fullest respect and affection.

"To the very close of his wonderful career he retained his accustomed health and vigor, as well as the possession, in their perfection, of all his faculties. No hand but his own can faithfully give us an account of the recreation and pleasure of that happy old age for which he entreats us all to strive. But we may sum it all up in the one brief line wherein he assures us: *'I never knew the world was beautiful until I reached old age!'*"

And Gualdo's description of Cornaro's passing sounds more like nature's kind intent than some of the deaths we currently read about. Gualdo wrote:

"When death came, it found him armed with the resignation of the philosopher and a steady courageous faith *in the future,* ready and glad to resign his life. Peacefully, as he had expected and foretold, he died at his palace in Padua, April 26, 1566, in the one hundred and third year of his age."

Cornaro had a positive approach truly remarkable in an age when sin, penance, and suffering were stressed—he also had a cheerful trust in the goodness of God. To me, as I think of approaching the Golden Age, I treasure these two paragraphs in his own words which come at the conclusion of his treatise on The Art of Living Long, written in his ninety-fifth year.

"Since some of them (holy men) believe that these afflictions are sent them by the great God for their salvation—that they may, in this life, make reparation for their sins—I cannot refrain from saying that, according to my judgment, these persons are mistaken; for I cannot believe God deems it good that man, whom He so much loves, should be sickly, melancholy, and discontented. I believe, on the contrary, that He wishes him to be healthy, cheerful, and contented, precisely as those holy men in ancient times were; who, becoming ever better servants of His Majesty, performed the many and beautiful miracles of which we read.

"In conclusion, I wish to say that, since old age is—as, in truth, it is—filled and overflowing with so many graces and blessings, and since I am one of the number who enjoy them, I cannot fail—not wishing to be wanting in charity—to give testimony to the fact, and to fully certify to all men that my enjoyment is much greater than I can now express in writing. I declare that I have no other motive for writing but my hope that the knowledge of so great a blessing as my old age has proved to be, will induce every human being to determine to adopt this praiseworthy orderly and temperate life, in favor of which I ceaselessly keep repeating, Live, live, that you may become better servants of God!" *

* *The Art of Living Long*—A new and improved English version of the treatise by the celebrated Venetian centenarian—Luigi Cornaro. Milwaukee, William F. Butler. 1914.

Chapter 21

❧❧❧❧❧❧

Turkey with a Ribbon

Do you know what happens to one turkey in a flock of turkeys if you put a red ribbon 'round its neck?

I've been told that the other turkeys immediately start to peck it to death.

The reason?

Well, a turkey with a red bow tie is "different"—and the "flock" will feel safer if this revolutionary is eliminated somehow.

Now, way back when we first met at the beginning of this book (a couple of million proteins ago!) I shared with you one of my favorite quotes by Max Mueller: "All truth is safe and nothing else is safe, and he who withholds truth from man for motives of profit or expediency is either a coward or a criminal or both."

But the world answers that with a question, the same question Pilate asked Jesus—"What is truth?"

Fortunately for you and me, a dedicated group of specialists and interested laymen are constantly trying to answer this as it relates to the science of Health; to your well-being and mine.

And when any among them believe he or she has discovered a truth that is not in line with current thinking, it takes great courage to bring it before the world.

Why?

Because, very often, such a one is held up to mockery, is often labeled crack-pot or quack, if nothing worse.

Again why?

Because he is a "turkey with a ribbon" charged with trying to install a new order or upsetting the status quo. When Louis Pasteur first advanced his germ theory of disease it was labeled by an important colleague as "a ridiculous fiction" and later his anthrax vaccine (the rediscovery of the vaccination technique which has since saved millions of lives) was viewed with doubt and mistrust, and his opponents ridiculed him with such statements as, "The microbe alone is pure and Pasteur is its prophet." Charles Darwin, upon publication of his "Origin of the Species," heard his work denounced as an "utterly rotten fabric of guess and speculation," and himself referred to as "an inhaler of mephitic gas."

It is perfectly right and just that the "new discovery" should come under careful scrutiny because there certainly *are* such things as quacks, frauds, materially-motivated health peddlers who prey on the desperation of the diseased and the gullability of the uninformed, as well as the sincere, but disappointing theorist who comes up with a "truth" that turns out to be no truth at all.

What separates the "true" from the "false" in such cases is careful investigation, scientific experimentation, and a bulk of evidence—or proof. And the great concern of some of us who are interested in the various aspects of the science of health—medicine, nutrition, bio-chemistry, psychology, improved farming methods, physical education, et al—is not so much that the discoverer of a "truth" will withhold it through cowardice (most of them will accept all manner of ridicule for their beliefs) or that the quack will "put one over" for profit or gain (many existing agencies attempt to protect the public on this score) as that the truth will flash as brightly as the turkey's red ribbon on a closed-minded flock who prefer the status quo—and disappear temporarily to be "re-discovered" at a later time (and truth always is re-discovered by the very nature of its existence) with a lot of the flock failing to get the benefits in the interim.

Several years ago, we established the Cummings Research Foundation, a medical and agricultural research foundation, primarily dedicated to researching the relationship between nutrition and the degenerative diseases, but interested (as this book no doubt indicates) in many ramifications designed to benefit humanity.

For instance we have supported the following projects:

At UCLA researching the growing of cheap protein food for animals as well as humans under the supervision of Dr. David Appleman of the Department of Irrigation and Soil Science, College of Agriculture.

At the Midwest Research Institute, Kansas City Missouri, researching the aging process under the supervision of Dr. Charles Kimball and Dr. William B. House.

At the Nutrition Laboratory of Fairleigh Dickinson University, Rutherford, New Jersey, researching cancer and applied nutrition, under the direction of Dr. Peter Sammartino and Dr. William E. Smith.

And we maintain a 400 volume nutritional reference library, the result of 40 years of research by Dr. Barnett Sure, formerly head of the Department of Agricultural Chemistry, University of Arkansas.

Proper research is very scientific and conclusions take a long time to reach.

For myself, personally, I've always found investigating the "turkey with the red or pink or green bow tie" equally fascinating, a sort of detective adventure, and very often rewarding. I've enjoyed studying their personalities. But I, personally, have never attempted to render a verdict. I won't do so now.

However, exciting things are always happening in this wonderful world and sometimes the strangest results come from the most unlikely sources. Take, for instance, the case of a small orphan boy who, one night heard his aunt say to his uncle, "You hear that boy's cough? He's got what his mother had; the doctor says he's not many more months for this world." Yet this same boy lingered long enough to observe his 83rd birthday by parachuting 2,500 feet into the Hudson River, declaring that old age is "just a bad habit." Between these two events he had changed the health habits of thousands of people and amassed a fortune as a publisher. He was most certainly a "turkey with a ribbon" (maybe two or three ribbons) and his name was Bernarr Macfadden.

Rebel with a Cause

Bernarr Macfadden was perhaps the world's most flamboyant exponent of the rugged life. He made a "fad" of nature, was called a crank and a quack; was called a healer and a savior, and only time and a mass of evidence has finally brought him into perspective as a pioneer in a good many health fields. It has not deprived him, however, of the label of the "rugged rebel" which his dramatic presentations of his beliefs earned for him.

Born in 1868, Macfadden was a "self-made" man—both physically and financially. After he overheard the doctor's prediction for his future—death in a few months from tuberculosis, the small boy decided to fight for life alone—his way. He scrounged dumbbells and exercise booklets and, weak as he was, he obeyed the instructions he read, and grew stronger. The coughing stopped. Eventually he was strong enough to run away from his uncle's farm. One of the odd jobs young Macfadden took was selling an exercise apparatus. He noticed that people liked the booklet he'd put out about the contraption better than the exerciser itself so he started Physical Culture Magazine, which soon gained a large following.

He believed, far in advance of his time, that proper diet, juices, fresh fruits, vegetables, nuts, whole grains, and meat, plus proper living habits and physical exercise, could cure many of man's health problems and he used his magazine to do battle for his beliefs.

As he had built himself from a sickly child into a hardy physical specimen, so in the early years of the 20th century he built his exercise pamphlet into a publishing empire, including not only magazines but a string of newspapers.

He still used his publications, particularly Physical Culture, to continue his health crusades. He boldly printed the facts about venereal disease, one of the first publishers to dare to put the facts before the public. He campaigned against patent medicines which, in those days, were claiming to cure anything from cancer to housemaid's knee. He believed that white flour was devitalizing the nation's basic diet and when, in the 1940s the makers of white bread began "enriching" their product, many interpreted this as a surrender to Macfadden's campaign.

A vegetarian during a part of his career (one of his favorite dishes was chopped carrots smothered in cottage cheese), he later began eating meat and was particularly fond of hamburger which he would eat with a variety of half-cooked vegetables. He believed that most people eat far too much, and that the body, when allowed to do so, could heal itself of many diseases by its own natural methods; and that any person, with enjoyment of all his powers, can prolong his life far beyond normal probabilities.

Macfadden further stated that the best foods are often the cheapest and, before the Second World War loomed, proved his point by showing Mussolini how he could cut his army's food bills and give Italy stronger soldiers. Macfadden was given a consignment of troops on which to experiment. Immediately he banned heavy starchy meals and crammed them instead with cracked wheat and "rabbit vegetables," meanwhile putting the men through calisthenics. So successful was he that he received an Italian decoration—which later, when these troops became embroiled against America, he threw away.

Macfadden was nothing if not controversial and most of his beliefs he expressed in the form of pet dislikes. He disliked high heels, skinny women, and corsets. As a matter of fact he reputedly paid his daughters not to wear "unhealthy, confining" under-garments, which stopped breath and circulation and were giving the fashionable women of that day the "vapors." He also inspired a "scandalous" public demonstration in which females "liberated" themselves of binding underthings and openly courted arrest by appearing with the "liberated women" who wore bloomers and middy blouses right on New York's public streets.

Despite ridicule from the status quo department, Macfadden built an enormous following which he converted to "nature's ways" and personally proved the worth of many of his crusades. Some, such as sleeping on the bare floor from his 67th year on, because he maintained that a hard floor is a strengthener of the spine, which he thought of as the center of human vitality have been neither proven nor generally accepted (for which I am grateful since I like a comfortable bed). Nor has his preference for women going barefooted ever taken hold (ditto!).

But without doubt he proved in his own life, in a somewhat spectacular fashion, not only by having nine children and three successive wives (the last of whom was 43 when he married her at the age of 80), not only by parachuting into the Hudson at 83, but by passing a flier's examination and continuing to pilot his plane after his 80th birthday, continuing to play a fast game of tennis, taking long hikes in winter storm or summer heat, and jumping over chair-backs practically 'til the moment of his death at 87, that wilting old age was a "bad habit." He could sustain his theory that the body, when allowed to do so by proper diet and proper physical care, had natural methods for sustaining health (he had not needed the services of a physician during his long and rugged life) and that nature's way was closer to fact than fad.

I didn't know Bernarr Macfadden well but met him briefly several times. His position as a physical culture pioneer seems unique to me—unique and colorful. *Very* colorful.

He was a rebel with a cause, a turkey who wore his red ribbon jauntily despite the attacks of the flock, stuck by his guns firing volley after volley and in the end achieved not only the obvious notoriety his methods evoked, but constructive reforms in many fields as well.

Gentleman Farmer

I met Louis Bromfield in 1940, gained an enormous respect for him, and watched his pioneer efforts with interest until the day of his death in 1956.

Bromfield was as different from Bernarr Macfadden in his aims, interests, and methods as it was possible to be. And yet both were men with a consuming passion for personal experimentations and, in their various ways, for making life better for you and me.

At 37, Louis Bromfield was one of the most distinguished writers in America. He had gained his reputation with such novels as "The Green Bay Tree" and won the Pulitzer Prize at the age of 30 for his "Early Autumn."

But Bromfield had a second interest beside literature. Born on a farm in Ohio, he originally chose farming as a profession and entered Cornell University School of Agriculture. Then he got to thinking and recalled "the poverty, hard work and narrow environment which then existed on the farm" and transferred to Columbia where he studied art. Before he could graduate, World War I broke out and he joined the French army as an ambulance driver. He never returned to college. Instead he lived in Europe during the 1920s. While he was writing he was also doing a little farming and gardening in the "old country," and a lot of thinking and dreaming.

In 1933 he bought a large farm in Lucas, Ohio, near his

birthplace and before many years had passed he and his family had settled on his farm, which he called "Malabar" after the Indian coastal region in his later successful novel, "The Rains Came."

Now his dream forced him into the role of pioneer. He divided his time between writing and farming—and his farming ideas, at first, made the neighboring farmers laugh—but the ridicule decreased as he began to put them into practice. Neighbors warned him that 99 per cent of Malabar was untillable. However, Bromfield started with what he called a "garden." His experiments centered around the observation that there were many plagues and blights and insect pests in America that he hadn't encountered in the Old Country. He said: "In all the years I farmed or gardened in the rich country of northern France we had never used a dust or an insecticide or a spray against either disease or insect pests. Why should there be so many plagues and insects here at home?" Many of the new forms of poisons put on the market each year to protect apples, celery, cabbage, string beans, etc., must somehow reach the people in residue form, he was convinced. He had equally strong feelings about chemical fertilizers. "Could it be," he asked himself, "that they are in part at least responsible for the increasing toll of heart disease, glandular derangements, cancer?"

In 1940, twenty years ago, I was on tour with Louella Parsons and a troupe making personal appearances. We were in Cleveland, Ohio, and after our evening show we went into a night club. Louis Bromfield, a friend of Louella's, was our host. He'd invited Louella with her whole company which consisted of about ten or twelve stars and starlets, for dinner.

Right there, in the night club, he gave us a little lecture on some of his theories. It was kind of a funny stage setting for that kind of a talk but we were all of us, Binnie Barnes, her husband, Mike Frankovitch, Bill Orr, Ilona Massey, Virginia O'Brien, June Priesser and the rest of the troupe, fascinated. Bromfield maintained that the sprays and other "patent medicines" were used mainly for the benefit of plants that were weak and unhealthy. Healthy plants don't get attacked by pests, he insisted. "Perhaps the truth is that our soils are depleted or minerally unbalanced?" He resolved to practice PREVENTIVE rather than PATENT medicine on his plants and soils. His New Agriculture consisted of working WITH nature rather than against her as so many farmers in the past had done.

He talked about his theory and his interest in soil conservation and he had the mark of the true crusader, a giant enthusiasm that made us all attentive.

Another spark that had inflamed the inspiration of Louis Bromfield in the field of agricultural experimentation was the now well-documented history of the Hunza, a tiny isolated nation existing and thriving for centuries between Kashmir and Pakistan high in the forbidding crags of the Himalayas.

Bromfield knew, as did Sir Robert McCarrison and many other highly reputable nutritional research scientists, that the fact that absolutely no disease existed or ever occurred among these hardy centenarians was a direct result of the national credo, "All that has come from the soil must go back, including you."

I was the only one among them, twenty years ago, who had had a little experience and a lot of interest in nutrition and I remember having a feeling that Bromfield, like my dad, was in advance of his time.

To begin to practice his theories of soil and plant improvement he used quantities of barnyard manure to supply organic material and a great many minerals as well as the animal secretions about which not much was then known.

"I knew the virtues of barnyard manure in making healthy plants," he said, "and I observed among other things that old farm gardens which had been manured and cultivated year after year in the same spot in Europe raised healthy vegetables which rarely if ever fell victims of disease or insects. This was so, very likely because for years the fertility and the minerals from the fields of the farm had been carried in through the manure and concentrated upon the small area of the garden. That soil had been fed constantly and the proper mineral balance had been maintained at the expense of the outlying fields which like our pasture had gradually become depleted."

Soon, Bromfield said, his plants were doing very well indeed. Insects could actually be seen around the healthy plants, but they did not attack. This was proved with peppers, eggplant, lettuce, and the whole range of root vegetables. Tomatoes and celery also were raised successfully under this method, and cabbage, too.

Bromfield held that two other procedures helped establish his basic method at Malabar. First, was the use by occasional irrigation of water from an old pond with a heavy population of fish which received, in times of heavy rains, run-off water from a neighboring barnyard. The richness of the pond (the trillions of tiny aquatic organisms spread over the garden) actually turned the water into a solution of weak fertilizer with a very nearly perfect mineral balance.

Second, he used mulch for nearly all vegetables. Whenever the mulch was lifted, it could be seen that fungi and moulds were attacking it and coverting it into organic material to feed the plants. And earthworms were attracted, spreading plant food throughout the soil and aerating the soil as well. The mulch used was wheat or oat straw or alfalfa hay or old pea vines. It varied, since Bromfield was especially careful not to introduce too much nitrogen and thus upset the natural mineral balance of the soil.

Later Bromfield summed up his Malabar procedures: "Immunity to some disease created through inoculation and the corrective effects of antibodies like penicillin and streptomycin in the case of disease are both well established, but no research has yet determined why balanced *health* should establish resistance and even immunity to disease in plants, animals and people."

For years after that first meeting I followed Louis Bromfield's activities and read of his progress and conclusions. One quote I remember distinctly. After many years at Malabar he said:

"In all of these fields of research there lie immense possibilities, revolutionary not only in the field of medicine and plant pathology, but in the field of life itself and the principles which determine the facts of life as well as the facts of decay, illness, and death. It is not only that in a cubic foot of good, living soil lies the pattern of the universe but that there may lie within it the key to that force which animates all living, growing things and establishes the difference between them and that which is inanimate and dead."

Bromfield was concerned with vigorous health for plants *and* people. He believed that his research and experimenting had effects on the whole aspect of health and even on the philosophies of dentists and doctors. And I believe that time is proving him correct.

For today the subject of the advantages of organic or "natural" farming and the possibility of ill-effect from sprays is now receiving careful investigation, intelligent experimentation and study in many quarters so that a "bulk of evidence" may bring to light the truth, whatever it is, for the benefit of humanity.

One interesting outgrowth has been the study of "natural" food supplements or those supplements which have a natural or organic source.

The research of supplements themselves has been more and more spotlighted. Many professional men and agencies which are dedicated to our protection and well-being have become concerned of late at the public's indiscriminate "dosing" with their potency vitamins.

Many uninformed people in the past few years have mistakenly arrived at the conclusion that high potency should be the determining factor in selecting an effective food supplement. "The higher the number, the better for me," they say. That's like the motion picture of a few years ago. A producer assumed that if one comedian made a comedy funny, five comedians would make it five times as funny, but often a tragedy was the result.

As one well-known nutrional scientist phrased the potency problem, the vitamin, the mineral, the enzyme are sparks. It takes very little of the right kind to do the job.

Or as you or I might say, "Why use a blow torch to light the furnace when a match will do?"

If high potency dosage is required your physician should be the one to diagnose the need and recommend whatever is necessary. Under normal conditions my medical friends feel it would be much more nutritionally sound if each person arrived at his highest efficiency by faithfully eating a daily dietary maintenance supplement of moderate or low potency.

Interestingly enough (and I'd like to think that this is partially the result of the crusading of my friend Bromfield) many of these professional men add "food supplements of moderate or low potency and *natural source*."

I think Louis would have liked that and would feel that 15 years after his death, his research and experiments were having a continuing effect.

I shall be eternally grateful to a great lady, Louella Parsons, for the many great people of our time whom she has caused me to meet, but few can rank higher in my esteem than Louis Bromfield.

Louis Bromfield, Pulitzer Prize winning author and Gentleman Farmer, was a man who willingly wore the red ribbon, was willing to be "different," was willing to court ridicule and misunderstanding, even becoming interested in politics from a farmer's point of view, to focus attention on the connection between farming procedures and the science of health.

~~~~~~

Chapter 22

Take Care of You — For Me

We have been asking how best to stay young, vital, energetic, attractive, useful for a full span of life.

And the answer seems to be that the truth about taking the *best* care of that remarkable tri-unity, our body, mind, and spirit, is still to find nature's laws and stick with this.

Bernarr Macfadden crusaded for "making a fad of nature." Louis Bromfield pioneered for a return to "natural farming."

But no crusader, no instructor, no expert, can *live* the answer for you or me. It's up to us.

I promised in the beginning of the book to share my experience and adventures with you—and I've done this faithfully—from tongue-grooves and proteins through vegetarianism. This chapter is a "detective detour" away from the main theme and it is offered simply to show you that the records are never closed on the sciences of health. Something new is always popping up to be proved or disproved. The adventures continue.

But in the simple program for Positive Health and Positive Living and Positive Thinking that I've outlined in the earlier chapters, I've kept my promise. I promised you from my own experience *that living the program changed my life—and can change yours.*

That if I could remember and apply it—so can you.

That if I have time to follow it—you do, too.

That, unless you have a specific medical problem, which must be treated by a medical specialist, *you can be your age and proud of it, whether you are thirty, or forty, or fifty, or sixty, active, attractive, vital, by living the rules we outlined.*

The time to start on this simple program of living is right now! *This* day.

I promised to observe the advice given by the King to the White Rabbit in Alice's Wonderland, to "begin at the beginning, and go on till you come to the end: then stop."

Well, we've come to the end. I've told you how I believe we can all be whole, wholesome, vital, beings—Man-As-Man-Should-Be. I have shown you how it has worked for me. I know it can work for you.

But *do* it. *Live* it. Try that Divine selfishness—because, remember, you have to *take care of you—for me!*

Acknowledgments

Elaine St. Johns, for her wonderful and talented collaboration.

My wife, Mary, and our brood, Bob, Melinda, Patricia, Laurie and Tony—the healthiest human guinea pigs I know.

Art Linkletter, who introduced book authorship into my life.

Rosalie Montgomery, who typed and typed and typed and typed.

Jerry Zeitman of Music Corporation of America, who has large shoulders, a kind heart, and infinite patience. On this project he read and read and read and read.

Motion Picture Director, Eddie Rubin ("Uncle Eddie" at our house), also a guinea pig and convert.

My dear friend, Milton Berle, for his positive approach to good health.

Edward L. Kramer, of the Kimball Foundation, St. Louis, Missouri, for the inspiration of his life as well as his writings.

Frank J. Hale, founder of the American Society for the Aged. For supplying great encouragement and research material.

Dr. David Appleman, of the Department of Irrigation and Soil Science, College of Agriculture, U.C.L.A.

Dr. O. B. Garrison, Director, South Carolina Agricultural Experimental Station, Clemson Agricultural College, South Carolina.

Dr. Howard H. Hillerman, Professor of Development Anatomy, Oregon State University, Corvallis, Oregon.

Dr. Charles Kimball, Midwest Research Institute, Kansas City, Missouri.

Dr. Peter Sammartino, President and Dr. William E. Smith, Directors of Nutritional Research, Fairleigh Dickinson University, Rutherford, New Jersey.

Dr. Barnett Sure, formerly head of the Department of Agricultural Chemistry, University of Arkansas, Fayetteville, Arkansas.

And to my dedicated and sincere friends in the nutritional world:

J. Earl Shooff
Rich Schnackenberg
Harry Ebbert
James Lewis
Paul Watson
W. C. Mainwaring
Leo Rhodifer
Dr. Dean Conrad

As well as the many other dedicated men and women whom I have never met, but who have shared their best efforts with me between book covers.

Selected Bibliography

E. M. Abrahamson, M.D. and A. W. Pezet, *Body, Mind and Sugar*,
Henry Holt and Company, New York, 1951.

U. S. Anderson, *Three Magic Words*,
Thomas Nelson & Sons, Toronto, New York, Edinburgh, 1954.

The American Journal of Clinical Nutrition,
Published by The American Journal of Clinical Nutrition, Inc., 49 W. 45th
St., New York City.

Dr. Allen E. Banik and Renee Taylor, *Hunza Land, The Fabulous Health
and Youth Wonderland of the World*,
Long Beach, California, Whitehorn Publishing Company.

Luigi Cornaro, *The Art of Living Long*,
A new and improved version of the Treatise by the Celebrated Venetian
Centenarian,
William F. Butler, Milwaukee, 1914.

Adelle Davis, *Let's Cook It Right*,
Harcourt Brace & Co., 1947.

Paul de Kruif, in collaboration with Rhea de Kruif, *Life Among the Doctors*,
Harcourt, Brace and Company, New York, 1949.

Catharyn Elwood, *Feel Like a Million*,
The Devin-Adair Company, 1956.

Lelord Kordel, Sc.D., *Eat and Grow Younger*,
The World Publishing Company, 1952.

Edward L. Kramer, *Pathways to Power*,
Kimball Foundation Press, St. Louis, Missouri, 1955.

Richard Mackarness, *Eat Fat and Grow Slim*,
Doubleday & Company, Inc., 1959.

Fred D. Miller, D.D.S., F.I.C.D., *Open Door to Health*,
The Devin-Adair Company, 1959.

Melvin E. Page, D.D.S., *Degeneration-Regeneration*,
Page Foundation, Inc., 1949.

Melvin E. Page, D.D.S., and D. L. Brooks, A.B., *Body Chemistry in Health and Disease,*
Page Foundation, Inc., 1954.

Neville, *Awakened Imagination,*
The G. & J. Publishing Co., 1954.

Weston A. Price, M.S., D.D.S., F.A.C.D., *Nutrition and Physical Degeneration,*
The American Academy of Applied Nutrition, 1939.

Margaret Rombauer, *The Joy of Cooking,*
Irma S. Rombauer and Marion Rombauer Becker,
The Bobbs-Merrill Co., Inc., 1953.

G. T. Wrench, M.D. (Lond.), *The Wheel of Health,*
Reprinted 1954 by Lee Foundation for Nutritional Research, Milwaukee, Wisconsin.
Originally printed by the C. W. Daniel Company Ltd., London, 1938.